HISTAMINE INTOLERANCE EXPLAINED

12 STEPS TO BUILDING A HEALTHY LOW HISTAMINE LIFESTYLE, FEATURING THE BEST LOW HISTAMINE SUPPLEMENTS AND LOW HISTAMINE DIET

TONY WRIGHTON

ABOUT THE AUTHOR

Tony Wrighton is a journalist and author, and he's histamine intolerant (though that's not how he introduces himself at parties.) His health and mindset-related books have now been published in 13 languages. He's also a broadcaster, regularly appearing on TV in the UK and globally.

DISCOVER MORE

Explore Tony's other titles, ranging from a bestselling histamine intolerance cookbook to fresh perspectives on health and mindset.

Histamine Intolerance Cookbook: Delicious, Nourishing, Low-Histamine Recipes, And Every Ingredient Labeled For Histamine Content

Beat Burnout: Overcome Exhaustion, Minimize Stress, and Take Back Your Life in 30 Days

Stop Scrolling: 30 Days to Healthy Screen Time Habits (Without Throwing Your Phone Away)

Learn NLP: Master Neuro-Linguistic Programming (the Non-Boring Way) in 30 Days

LEGAL & DISCLAIMER

The information contained in this book is not designed to replace or take the place of any form of medicine or professional medical advice. The information in this book has been provided for educational and entertainment purposes only.

You need to consult a professional medical practitioner in order to ensure you are both healthy enough and able to make use of this information. Always consult your professional medical practitioner before undertaking any new dietary regime, and particularly after reading this book.

The information contained in this book has been compiled from sources deemed reliable, and it is accurate to the best of the Author's knowledge; however, the Author cannot guarantee its accuracy and validity and cannot be held liable for any errors or omissions.

Upon using the information contained in this book, you agree to hold harmless the Author, and Publisher, from and against any damages, costs, and expenses, including any legal fees potentially resulting from the application of any of the information provided by this guide. This disclaimer applies to any damages or injury caused by the use and application, whether directly or indirectly, of any advice or information presented, whether for breach of contract, tort, negligence, personal injury, criminal intent, or under any other cause of action. You agree to accept all risks of using the information presented inside this book.

CONTENTS

WHAT TO EXPECT

In this book, I offer a comprehensive approach to understanding and managing histamine intolerance. Supported by the very latest research, this guide offers an effective program and mindset shift towards healing.

In Chapters 1-3, I unpack the basics of histamine and address what, for many, is an unanswered question: Do You Really Have Histamine Intolerance? I share my journey of living with histamine intolerance for over 20 years, before it was recognized by conventional medicine, and I look at the science behind this condition.

Then we get into the good stuff; a 30-day low-histamine program, offering practical suggestions on how to make effective changes in the area of diet, supplements and lifestyle and finding a practitioner.

Chapter 4 is an exploration of the Low-Histamine Diet. We dive into the foods you want to avoid, the dishes you can enjoy, and the essentials you should always have in your kitchen. It's not just about restriction; it's about finding delicious and nourishing alternatives that won't aggravate your histamine intolerance.

Chapter 5 is all about a Histamine-Healing Mindset. I focus on the power of rest and reflection – a crucial part of the puzzle. If you're like me, your inclination may be to skip this bit. "Yeh, sure, mindfulness and all that". Please give it a chance though. The scientifically-proven links between stress and histamine intolerance may surprise you. Without calming your body and mind down, you won't heal properly.

In **Chapter 6**, I focus on a Low-Histamine Lifestyle. Factors such as the air we breathe, our living conditions, electromagnetic fields, and even seemingly minor details such as moisture and humidity can affect our body's histamine levels. I also examine supplements and medication and how they can help us on our low-histamine journey.

In **Chapter 7,** I venture into advanced territory. I guide you through finding a healthcare practitioner who is experienced in histamine intolerance and review some of this field's most advanced questions. Oh, and there's a deep dive into histamine intolerance + coffee (because *everyone* asks about coffee!)

Then in **Chapters 8-11**, you'll find my 'Low-Histamine Survival Kit': a detailed ingredient list designed to simplify your grocery shopping, as well as food polls, histamine-friendly products and services, and even a 30-Day Histamine Intolerance Symptom Tracker. This will allow you to document your symptoms, identify potential triggers, and better understand your body's unique responses. This Survival Kit aims to be your one-stop guide to not just surviving but thriving on a low-histamine lifestyle.

And finally **Chapter 12** is all about the future – one that is healthy and low histamine.

Before we jump into all that, let's rewind to a time when histamine intolerance had a significant impact on my life...

INTRODUCTION

If you're reading this book, the chances are that something feels off. Maybe you have constant gut symptoms, bloating, wind, or stomach discomfort. Perhaps you have unexplained issues with your skin. Or, you might have the classic allergy symptoms of a runny nose and itchy eyes – but all year round. Perhaps your symptoms are more serious, connected to inflammation, hormones or extreme fatigue. Maybe you can't pigeonhole your symptoms and your illness. *Something is just not quite right.*

That was me for many years. Something felt off.

What Happened on My Wedding Night

It was a joyous occasion at a beautiful hotel by the sea in a remote part of the UK called Cornwall.

After a beautiful, intimate ceremony with just our infant son and two witnesses, we celebrated all day and evening. Everything was perfect. Our son even fell asleep in minutes (rather than the normal torturous two-hour toddler bedtime), so we could carry on celebrating.

But as bedtime approached, I noticed something that nobody wants to notice on their wedding night.

I know you're probably thinking: What on earth will he say? What wedding night bedtime revelations could possibly merit inclusion in this book?

Histamine intolerance wreaks its havoc in many ways, which are unique to each person. For example, I get a blocked nose when I eat chocolate. My belly reacts to pineapple. And my unwelcome wedding night revelation was that I had developed a rather unattractive and irritating rash over the course of the evening.

I'd never been married before, so I'd never worn a wedding ring. And when I put my wedding ring on, or rather when my new wife put it on me, my body reacted to it. It turns out my skin reacts to certain metals in jewelry. As I know now, this is not uncommon, but it didn't make me feel any less self-conscious at the time. The gold in the ring was mixed with a small amount of nickel, and nickel reactions are quite common in people with histamine intolerance. Hence the rash.

Initially, this tiny rash was on my finger and hand, but it was a bit less tiny the next day. It had spread to different parts of my body.

Oh, joy!

My first day of married life, and look at me. My hands and feet were now covered. After a couple of days and a process of elimination, I realized that the wedding ring might be the problem.

Ring Of Fire

Research shows that nickel in jewellery is the most common cause of skin contact issues – for example, this applied to approximately 16% of patch-tested dermatology patients in Germany. (1) In the specific instance of histamine intolerance, the immune response can misinterpret nickel as a threat, which was what led to my unpleasant wedding ring skin rash.

Interestingly, the use of nickel in jewelry is restricted by law in Britain and the EU due to its allergenic nature, but not so in the US, where we had happened to buy the rings. It was something I thought was special and loving, but that turned out to be a "rash" decision. (Not my last Dad joke!)

So, having spent a reasonable amount on a wedding ring, I took it off two days after getting married. It is now gathering dust in a drawer somewhere. We are still happily married, but I'm a happily married non-ring-wearer. I wore a $3 silicone ring for a bit. But understandably, my wife wasn't that keen. Other options include platinum or stainless steel, which are hypoallergenic, or I could have got the ring "dipped" in platinum. Alternatively, I suggested to my wife that I could get a ring tattoo instead – again, she wasn't that keen!

Episodes like this showed me how seemingly random or minor aspects of daily life could unexpectedly contribute to histamine intolerance symptoms. The realization that there is so much more beneath the surface inspired me to dive deeper and share what I've learned about managing this condition.

The Story So Far

This book and its sister title, *Histamine Intolerance Cookbook*, were originally published under my company name, Ketoko Guides. This was a name adopted for my specialized series of health books. The idea was to allow me to work with a small team and specifically address an audience interested in health and nutrition. This differed a bit from my previous books, where I've been fortunate to have some success.

There was only one problem with Ketoko Guides. Everyone knew it was me behind the books. The histamine intolerance world is small, and after all I made no secret of the fact that I'd published it with my talented team. So who was I trying to kid?

And there was another thing. For a number of years now, I've connected with a surprising number of individuals dealing with histamine intolerance through instagram and my website. Lots of people reach out every single day, frustrated because their practitioners just don't 'get' histamine intolerance—some even brush it off completely. I personally respond to these people and so I wanted to put my name to a new version of *Histamine Intolerance Explained*.

This edition is completely updated, refreshed, and expanded. It is an update that has been more than a year in the making and has seen me work with some of the best in the business. For this latest version, I've had the privilege of collaborating with industry leaders, including a distinguished health editor known for her work with renowned food and lifestyle brands.

I also thank the other editors and fact-checkers who have contributed to presenting you with this fresh new look at histamine intolerance. It's been a labor of love to update and I'm incredibly proud of it. I'd love you to give me any feedback and you can do that at www.tonywrighton.com.

Now that you've heard a bit of my story, next up is a quick quiz to see if you're part of the histamine intolerance club. (Admittedly, it's not the coolest club to be in, but hey, we're in it together.)

If you already know you're histamine intolerant and understand *The Invisible Battle*, you might also want to skip ahead to Part 2: *The Road To Recovery*. It's packed with the info you need to get started right away. Remember, Part 1 will always be here, going in-depth whenever you're ready to revisit it.

PART 1:

THE INVISIBLE BATTLE

1. Quiz: Do I Really Have Histamine Intolerance?

Some experts estimate that up to 17% of the population suffers from histamine intolerance. It's now time to see if you're among that number. Here's a quiz covering the myriad of symptoms you might expect with histamine intolerance – and the list is long.

That's why the whole first part of my book is entitled *The Invisible Battle*. There could be lots of stuff that has been going on for years that you've just now linked to histamine issues.

For instance, I'm a super sniffer: I have an extremely sensitive nose, and smells affect me big time. If I stand in a queue behind someone with a strong scent or perfume, I have to leave the shop; if a TV studio I am presenting in gets cleaned with bleach, I struggle to focus; we switch to a new (eco-friendly) rhubarb-scented cleaner, and it makes me gag. So, we can add sniffing to the long list of symptoms.

> *Figuring out histamine intolerance is like being a detective in your own body – every symptom is a clue.*

Here's the quiz. The symptoms start in quite generalized terms and then get more specific. Keep a note of your tally of As, Bs and Cs.

Please note that this quiz is intended as a guide for you to use with your practitioner. You can take more extensive tests for histamine intolerance, but they vary based on the time of the day, time of the month, what you had for breakfast, whether your body is fighting off an infection, and all sorts of other variables. Always consult your practitioner before starting any new dietary or wellness regime.

1. Do you get anxious - often without apparent reason?

  A) Rarely
  B) Sometimes
  C) Often

2. Do you experience shortness of breath, not necessarily linked to exercise?

  A) Never
  B) Sometimes
  C) Often

3. Do you notice your heart rate racing?

  A) Never
  B) Sometimes
  C) Often

4. Do you suffer from severe menstrual pain?

  A) No
  B) Yes, but it's manageable
  C) Yes, and it's severe

5. Do you feel exhausted or burnt out?

  A) Rarely
  B) Sometimes
  C) Often

6. Do you feel dizzy?

  A) Never

B) Sometimes
C) Often

7. Do you sneeze a lot?

A) Never
B) Sometimes
C) Often

8. Do you suffer from a runny or blocked nose? Are you sensitive to smells (in other words, are you a super sniffer like me)?

A) Never
B) Sometimes
C) Often

9. Do you get watery, itchy, or red eyes?

A) Never
B) Sometimes
C) Often

10. Do you suffer from headaches?

A) Never
B) Sometimes
C) Often

11. Do you experience sleep problems of any kind? These might include struggling to drop off, waking up in the middle of the night, waking up early, or sleeping poorly?

A) No, I sleep like a baby
B) Sometimes
C) Often, my sleep is terrible

12. Do you sometimes suffer from restless legs (Restless Leg Syndrome), characterized by jerky leg or body movements, particularly at night?

A) No
B) Yes, but it's manageable
C) Yes, and it's severe

14. Do you get cold hands and feet? Do you suffer from poor circulation?

A) No
B) Yes, a bit
C) Yes, a lot

15. Do you experience gut issues?

A) Never
B) Sometimes
C) Often

16. Do you have regular or sporadic diarrhea?

A) Never
B) Sometimes
C) Often

17. Do you suffer from bloating and gas?

A) Never
B) Sometimes
C) Often

18. Do you often feel nauseous without any apparent reason?

A) Never
B) Sometimes
C) Often

19. Do you experience inflammation anywhere in the body?

A) Rarely
B) Sometimes
C) Often

20. Do you suffer from skin issues? Dry skin, eczema, patchy stuff?

A) Never
B) Occasionally
C) Frequently

21. Do you suffer from hives, small red bumps, or itchy spots?

A) Never
B) Occasionally
C) Frequently

22. Do you suffer from constipation?

A) Never
B) Occasionally
C) Often

23. Have you been diagnosed with IBS (Irritable Bowel Syndrome)?

A) No
B) Yes, but it's under control
C) Yes, and it's often problematic

Scoring:

Every A) answer = 0 points
Every B) answer = 1 point
Every C) answer = 2 points

Results:

- **0-4 points:** Great news, you have scored low on this histamine intolerance test. But wait, it doesn't completely rule out the possibility that you might have histamine intolerance. Your symptoms may be milder, or just not covered in my (admittedly unscientific) quiz.
- **5-9 points:** You might have histamine intolerance. Yes I know this isn't the conclusive diagnosis you were hoping for, but hey, what did you expect from a quiz. The truth is, your symptoms do indicate that you may have histamine intolerance. Follow my program in Part 2: The Road To Recovery and see if your symptoms start to improve.
- **10 points and above:** You have scored highly for histamine intolerance symptoms. Obviously this is not an official diagnosis, but I suggest you follow Part 2: The Road To Recovery and monitor your symptoms to see if they improve.

Now that you've taken the test, read on to understand what histamine intolerance is and what it's doing to your body.

2. Histamine Intolerance 101 (and Why Is It So Under the Radar?)

"Health is not valued until sickness comes."

–Thomas Fuller

One month before the birth of my son, I was feeling weak, dizzy, and extremely anxious. There was plenty to be worried about (moving house, financial stress, and the impending arrival of a tiny human who would change my wife's and my lives forever). Naturally, I put this heightened state of anxiety down to the little ball of cuteness that was about to hit us, but there was more going on.

My health just wasn't right. I was suffering from an unpleasant and unattractive mix of symptoms: runny nose, uneasy/upset belly, low energy, and (worst of all!) a worsening intolerance to alcohol. My heart rate would often race (which is not pleasant), I was developing a particularly irritating "watery eye", and I'd tried everything.

Well, almost everything.

There was one condition left at the bottom of my list. I had yet to look into it in any great detail. Honestly, I was putting it off, as it seemed so complicated.

I had first heard about histamine intolerance years earlier at a health conference in California. I had gone to a lecture by someone I'd never heard of before: Dr Ben Lynch – who, as it turns out, is a brilliant and prominent doctor in the world of histamine. He mentioned histamine issues and how debilitating histamine intolerance could be. I whipped out my phone and asked Dr. Google. Words like histaminosis, basophils and diamine oxidase popped up. Waaay too confusing. I mentally filed histamine intolerance away under "just another crazy health concept that has nothing to do with me".

In the following years, I tried every other diet and approach, and nothing worked. Over the past decade, I've been lucky enough to meet some of the world's most famous and celebrated experts in the world of health, diet and wellness, while recording my podcast and writing my books. They all told me the same thing; while there are a number of rules that tend to work for most people, there is no perfect "one-size-fits-all" diet for everyone. We are all unique and have to find what suits us best. I explored:

- gluten-free
- dairy-free
- nut-free
- keto
- Paleo
- low oxalate
- low lectin
- and more (lots more!)

Don't judge me here. You're already judging me, aren't you? Oh well. Anyway, all of them had pros and cons. For example, I enjoyed Paleo; keto was fun, but I lost too much weight. I'm still happily gluten-free.

But none of these diets seemed to fully resolve my health issues.

The only diet left on my list was the one I'd heard of years earlier: Low Histamine. What the hell was that? I dimly remembered the histamine doctor I'd gone to see talking about the low-histamine diet years earlier at a biohacking conference in LA.

But every time I looked at it, it just seemed so mind-boggling. How could I possibly go shopping for low-histamine items without consulting Google every time?

You may well be the same. If you are, I'm here to hold your hand and make it as easy to understand as possible. That is why I've included a comprehensive food list and shopping list at the end of this book. If you're reading this in paperback and you'd rather have the list on your mobile, go to The Histamine Intolerance Site Food List (www.histamineintolerance.net/foodlist) and bookmark that page.

As a journalist, I'm passionate about providing quality information to you, which is a real challenge with histamine intolerance. There's no doubt – it's a tough one to explain. For a long time, I had to squint and think really hard when explaining it. So let's make it as accessible as we can. Let's start with a metaphor about a house party....

Party-Time

Picture your body as a house hosting a party, where histamine is represented by the guests (bear with me here!). In a healthy scenario, a moderate number of guests (just the right amount of histamine) ensures the party is enjoyable and functions well.

However, imagine if too many guests suddenly flood in, overcrowding the house. This is akin to an excess of histamine in your body, where the balance is disrupted and things start to go sideways. The music gets too loud, conversations turn into shouting matches, and the once-organized buffet becomes chaotic. The party (your body) gets out of control.

That's what's going on when you suffer from histamine intolerance. Some of us have an out-of-control party raging in our bodies, and it needs someone to come in and turn the music off!

We will tame this wild house party in the program in Part 2: *The Road To Recovery*. We'll ask the rowdy guests to leave and focus on maintaining histamine balance to keep the good times rolling without any unwanted chaos. (Okay, that's enough of the house party analogy...)

The Science Behind Histamine Intolerance

Histamine intolerance is what happens when your body has trouble breaking down histamine, a chemical involved in your immune system, digestion, and communication between your body and brain. (1, 2) You can't and wouldn't want to completely eliminate histamine, but when there's too much of it in your body, it can cause various symptoms. Those become uncomfortable and sometimes even severe. (1, 2)

Studies have demonstrated common symptoms of histamine issues, including; headaches, stomach pain, bloating, dizziness, and irregular heart rate. (1, 3) These symptoms can be similar to those associated with allergies, making it challenging to diagnose. (1, 2, 3, 4)

But histamine's reach is far and wide, affecting several critical organs, such as the cardiovascular system (heart palpitations, anyone?), lungs, gut, skin, and central nervous system (hello, anxiety). So, when your body can't break down histamine effectively, you find yourself grappling with histamine intolerance. And just like that house party, things get out of control.

So Why Is Histamine Intolerance Still So Under the Radar?

This is an excellent question. I have found an ever-increasing number of people coming to my site seeking answers. Despite much medical literature on histamine intolerance, it can be tricky to diagnose and treat, and people often spend years baffled by their symptoms and disease.

> "Health is a puzzle; sometimes the piece you're missing is not the most obvious."

Here are a few suggestions as to why it is still under the radar of many practitioners and the health world at large:

1. The list of histamine intolerance symptoms is long, and it often mimics those of other disorders and allergies. It's tough to pinpoint without a comprehensive examination (5). For instance, I had a dodgy gut for years, and, despite visits to top gastroenterologists in the country, they didn't pinpoint histamine issues.
2. Histamine intolerance varies massively between individuals. Some people react differently to identical

supplements and medications recommended for histamine issues. (3) I am extremely sensitive and have learned to take as little as a tenth of the recommended dose of any supplement or treatment when starting out. Many others report similar experiences. I empty the pills, divide them in half and pour the rest down the sink.

3. Histamine intolerance isn't definitively curable, since experts have yet to establish a clinical diagnosis. (6, 7, 8).

4. Conventional allergy tests don't cut it for diagnosing histamine intolerance, as it's not an allergy as such. Some tests are available for histamine levels, but they're often unreliable. Practitioners often use a process of elimination to reach a conclusion (9), a method that can work well. That's what we'll be doing in the program in Part 2: *The Road To Recovery*.

We know histamine intolerance is complicated, and these factors are just some of the reasons why it is under the radar.

Histamine Intolerance: Emerging Perspectives

I wanted a medical perspective on why histamine issues are so under-appreciated, so I approached Dr. Tina Peers. She is a consultant specializing in menopause, mast cell activation and histamine intolerance. Most recently, she's developed a particular interest in helping patients deal with Long Covid, and has noticed how many have histamine intolerance symptoms.

We ended up having several illuminating conversations; here's what she told me about histamine intolerance being so under the radar:

"I don't blame doctors who haven't heard about it, or who don't know the latest findings or discoveries. It's a very early science. There's an awful lot to learn; there's an awful lot yet to be discovered... We think as much as 17% of the population has a problem with their mast cells, and so it's terribly, terribly common. Therefore, there's a large proportion of people in the population who are struggling in one way or another at various times in their lives, or throughout their whole lives, and they need help. So, yes, I think we need to shine a light on it a bit more."

The thought of a large number of individuals enduring symptoms "throughout their whole lives" disturbed me. Despite societal advances, we are still dealing with emerging perspectives, and our understanding of histamine intolerance is in its infancy.

Before I said goodbye to Dr. Tina, she told me the reason she had first become interested in histamine intolerance. Her daughter had suffered from a series of heartbreaking symptoms, even as a very young child. At the age of seven, she had developed angina – chest pain caused by reduced blood flow to the heart muscles. She had gone on to suffer from a whole host of symptoms that nobody wants to see their child go through (including hyperthyroid, extreme lethargy, unexplained headaches, eczema, and more besides).

At the time Dr. Tina had heard about histamine intolerance, but was not specializing in this area. Unfortunately, her daughter's health issues worsened as an adult. In her 20s, she decided to radically overhaul her diet and lifestyle. She wanted to prioritize her health, but, without realizing it, she was making her health even worse.

"Consuming large amounts of tomatoes, spinach, and avocados, all of which are generally healthy but harmful if one can't metabolize the histamine properly, only made her progressively sicker.

"I suspect she made smoothies packed with avocados and spinach, treating it like the miracle cure-all. At first, she thought she had the flu, but then she began to experience every symptom associated with high histamine. Fainting spells, severe dizziness, midnight nausea, intense Irritable Bowel Syndrome, facial swelling. There was a morning when she woke up, and her face had swollen so much it resembled a football. Her lips were so inflamed and cracked she could hardly drink water. It was dreadful.

"That was when we made the diagnosis. Distressed and in tears, she called me and shared how she couldn't touch her skin because of the excruciating pain. She was so sick and didn't know what was happening to her. Since she wasn't living at home at that time, I hadn't been able to notice her gradual deterioration. As soon as I heard her condition, I rushed over, brought her home, and that's when my husband pointed out how it seemed like she was reacting to everything. He suggested it might be histamine.

"Once he said the word 'histamine,' I looked up histamine intolerance again. This time, however, there was a lot more information compared to nine years earlier. That's when I made the diagnosis; she had histamine intolerance. This experience sparked my interest in the subject. And since

then, you can't unlearn something, can you? So once you know about something, you see it everywhere."

This story deeply resonated with me. Over the years, I had strived for health but ended up sicker. I, too, was loading up my shopping trolley with ingredients like avocado and spinach, yet that had been the worst thing I could have done.

I had been fighting the invisible battle. It was histamine all along.

Unearthing Hidden Answers

Discovering the truth about our health can be a journey of patience and persistence, especially when it comes to histamine intolerance. Just like digging for buried treasure, the real answers are often hidden beneath the surface, waiting to be uncovered.

I caught up with Dr. Tina about a year later, and she updated me. Her daughter was doing well on the low-histamine lifestyle and had just become a mother herself. She told me, "She's just one of the best mummies in the world. She's absolutely brilliant, completely devoted and besotted with her little one."

I was so pleased that Dr. Tina shared her story with me and my podcast listeners. It is a powerful testament to the transformative power of understanding our bodies and taking control of our health.

"Just try it for three days..."

Let's go back to one month before the birth of my boy. Despite having plenty on my plate, I was feeling rubbish enough to finally start to investigate this weird concept called histamine intolerance. I read online that I could just try a low-histamine diet for three days to see if I felt better.

In fact, I felt better within *hours*. It was an enormous change. I'm really not kidding here.

This is the potential magic of going low-histamine . It may take longer for you, and that's why I suggest a 30-day program in Part 2: *The Road To Recovery*. But, it might surprise you how quickly you will feel better. The body can start to clear that excess histamine relatively quickly.

Back then, as you know, I was struggling badly with a runny nose and eyes (attractive, huh) as well as a constant anxious feeling (very unpleasant) and the usual gut issues. Most of these issues immediately started to improve. It was such a relief.

However, my path to recovery wasn't a straight line. I remember eating a rich butterbean soup on the day my son was born and wincing through the birth. (I could hardly whine about a stomach ache when my wife was single-handedly redefining the phrase "pain scale" while welcoming our child into the world). But apart from the evil butter beans, my symptoms mainly started to improve rapidly.

I genuinely hope the same applies to you. The program in Part 2: *The Road To Recovery* will examine ways to fix histamine intolerance issues. It starts with diet (where my first, initial easy wins took place), and then we move to lifestyle, sleep, mindset, and supplements – all of which can also have a dramatic impact. But before that, let's understand your symptoms more deeply.

The Histamine Bucket

At this point, it's worth introducing the "Histamine Bucket" concept, which you will hear about repeatedly in the histamine intolerance world.

This concept was originally popularized by the brilliant author Janice Joneja, who introduced the idea that our tolerance for histamine can be imagined as our body having a histamine "bucket".

This bucket can only hold a certain amount of histamine at a time. When the bucket is low, you could eat all of the wrong foods, do all of the wrong things in terms of histamine, and you'll probably be okay. As long as the bucket doesn't overflow, everything is okay. You might not even notice your symptoms until the bucket overflows.

However, when it does overflow, you'll know about it! That might be why you're reading this book now.

I have found this to be true so many times on my own histamine journey. I can seem to eat all the wrong foods for months on end, but,when I'm having a histamine flare-up, I can just look at a piece of dark chocolate and feel terrible. The bucket is full to the brim, and when I add anything to it, the excess histamine spills into my system.

So that's the metaphor. Now you know what the histamine bucket is; over the next 30 days we'll work to keep it nice and low at all times.

3. Exploring the Root Cause: Exactly Why Are You Histamine Intolerant?

It's important to understand the 'why' behind your histamine intolerance, as this gives you crucial information for long-term healing. Histamine intolerance rarely appears out of the blue; something else is usually going on. So what might it be? There is a reason; we just need to figure it out.

Unraveling the reasons behind your histamine intolerance can take a while. At this point, I should probably admit that it took me more than 20 years, but don't let that put you off, as I didn't have this book to help.

Here are some of the potential contributors to histamine issues.

- Genes
- Gut imbalance
- Mold exposure
- Hormones
- Long Covid

This list is not exhaustive, but it's a start. Let's look at each one in more detail, and see if they apply to you. And as we go, you'll discover more about my own 'root cause'.

Genes

I stared at the piece of paper in front of me.

Complete gobbledygook. A jumble of seemingly random letters denoting various genetic markers that may or may not be linked to histamine intolerance.

MAO. DAO. COMT. MTHFR.

How was I going to make sense of this?

Sometimes, histamine intolerance is a genetic thing, and these confusing combinations of letters stand for certain genes that can impact histamine intolerance. Some people are just more genetically susceptible, so is your histamine intolerance hereditary?

It's a complicated and ever-developing area, so a good start is getting your genetics tested and consulting with a practitioner.

You can also crunch the data yourself. Trust me, I've tried. You may get bogged down in a sea of MAO, DAO, COMT, and MTHFR but it is possible.

Navigating Genetic Analysis: Picking the Right Site

Sites like 23andMe offer an attractive interface and easy user experience, but their fairly generic health analysis could offer more about histamine intolerance. What you have to do is extract the raw data and get a genetic report from a specialist provider. Here are two options I like:

> ◼ **Dr. Rhonda Patrick's Found My Fitness website**
> ◼ **Dr. Ben Lynch's Strategene site**
>
> **Both sites provide a much more complete report on your genetic predisposition to histamine intolerance.**

There is one gene which I want to go into in more detail on.

The DAO gene plays a crucial role in histamine intolerance. The DAO (diamine oxidase) enzyme helps to break down histamine in the gut. If you have histamine intolerance, the DAO enzyme may not be functioning properly or be present in insufficient quantities. This leads to our old friend, histamine intolerance. The DAO gene encodes the DAO enzyme, and variations in this gene have been linked to histamine intolerance.

I am histamine intolerant but do not have a variation in the DAO gene. This illustrates the fact that histamine intolerance is a complex condition. The DAO gene is just one of many factors that can contribute to it.

Research in this area is evolving all the time, and while you are better off speaking to a practitioner, it is often frustratingly expensive to find someone who can help you analyze your data.

DAO Supplements: Histamine's Little Helpers?

Since diamine oxidase is the primary enzyme responsible for breaking down ingested histamine, some people with histamine intolerance may have lower levels of this enzyme. If that's you, taking a DAO supplement may help you tolerate foods with histamine better. Don't expect these supplements to wear a cape and save the day single-handed, but they may well help with your histamine issues considerably. I cover these in Chapter 6 and also list some providers in the Low-Histamine Survival Kit section.

I approached histamine and MCAS expert Beth O'Hara to shed some more light on genetics. She told me our genes provide a blueprint for our bodies that gives clues to how we might react with histamine intolerance, but also that the presence of a particular gene does not provide a diagnosis.

"Our genetics are only a predisposition; it's like a blueprint for our bodies, but it's not diagnostic. These genes that we're looking at: they tell us where you have predispositions or weaknesses, and it's a big part of why people could have the same root causes. So, you'd have five people with Lyme and Mold toxicity, and they all present in a different way because it depends on our genetic predispositions, how things are expressed."

This goes back to my tests. You might not have any genetic tendency towards histamine intolerance and nonetheless still have it. Or you might have all the genes, but be absolutely 100% clear of it. It just provides an indicator, nothing more.

Conclusion: your best bet is to ask your histamine-knowledgeable practitioner to help you analyze your genetics and decide on a plan.

Gut imbalance

Histamine intolerance can often manifest because you've got an imbalance in your gut. This is thought to be primarily due to the critical role the gut plays in the regulation of histamine levels. Our gut microbiota, which consists of billions of bacteria, plays a pivotal role in breaking down histamine.

Sometimes, this is the fault of the pesky diamine oxidase (DAO), which we've already looked at. But it might not be genetic. As Dr. Ben Lynch (the bloke I watched at that conference all those years ago) pointed out, If you have small intestinal bacterial overgrowth (SIBO) or another form of gut imbalance, then perhaps histamine is the issue or the resultant cause. High levels of histamine are routinely found in patients with inflammatory bowel disease (IBD). (10)

But for me, while I was definitely suffering from stomach issues, there was a deeper underlying issue causing my histamine issues in the gut. In other words, it wasn't just SIBO.

Mold exposure

Most of us have heard about mold triggering allergic reactions, asthma attacks, and respiratory issues. However, previous mold exposure is considered a leading cause of histamine intolerance. A big problem with mold exposure is that you may not even realize it has happened. Sometimes mold is very obvious, but sometimes it's hiding behind a wall, ceiling or chimney and causing you problems. (11)

This mold exposure may not be current. It might have been a long time ago. You might be living in a lovely, dry, warm, cozy house with no mold now, but have suffered previous exposure and it's still affecting you. For example, I once lived in Florence, Italy. The flat I rented had a unique, musty smell. It was a beautiful old building, but how much mold was hiding behind those walls?

If there's a smell in a property that can be an indication something is not right. *There was definitely a smell.* If only I'd known that then.

But why is this an issue? Mycotoxins are toxic substances produced by mold. Prolonged mold exposure can lead to high mycotoxin levels in the body. This is the root cause of my own histamine intolerance. Studies have suggested that mycotoxins and histamine issues are linked. (12) Elevated histamine from mycotoxins can overwhelm our body's natural ability to break it down, leading to our old friend histamine intolerance.

Unfortunately, that's not all. High levels of mycotoxins lead to all sorts of issues in the body, and in some cases (such as aflatoxin) they are considered a carcinogen. This can become serious in the long term and needs to be addressed. You can see how seriously we want to take mycotoxins in the body.

So I can now trace the start of my health and histamine issues back to the time I lived in that flat with the funny smell. As I said before - if only I'd known.

We'll investigate this more in Chapter 6: *Low-Histamine Lifestyle*, when we clean up our environment. However, as I've found, if mold/mycotoxins are the source of your histamine intolerance, you will almost certainly need to commit to a healing process that lasts longer than 30 days.

Hormones

"Histamine and estrogen are linked – the number of mast cells, and the amount of histamine they produce, fluctuates throughout the menstrual cycle, rising as estrogen levels rise and falling as estrogen levels fall. Estrogen increases histamine levels by triggering mast cells to release their stored histamine and down-regulates DAO, the enzyme responsible for clearing excess histamine from the body."

Performanceinhealth.com

The dance between hormones and histamine in our bodies is intricate and complicated. I'll outline some key points, but, even after delving into this complex area for some time, I've found it remains a nuanced subject best tackled with the guidance of a true hormone health professional.

Menstrual Cycle Effects:

During ovulation and periods, many women seem to experience histamine-related changes. There are a number of potential factors here, including:

- Estrogen and Histamine: Estrogen levels rise and fall throughout the menstrual cycle. When they are high, they can spike histamine release. (13)
- Progesterone and Histamine: Progesterone levels also vary. Progesterone plays the opposite role. It can be a calming influence on histamine, telling it to take a break.

- DAO Enzyme Fluctuations: DAO, (that's the histamine-busting enzyme we covered earlier), doesn't stay constant. Its levels vary during different menstrual phases. This affects histamine breakdown. (14)

Pregnancy

It's worth briefly mentioning that, during pregnancy, many women experience a reduction in histamine intolerance symptoms. This is thought to be thanks to the natural increase in DAO production, which helps break down histamine more efficiently. Unfortunately, after they give birth, the DAO production seems to go back to its original level.

Menopause and Histamine:

Many women reaching out to me have said that their histamine issues worsen during menopause. It's thought that fluctuating estrogen levels can exacerbate histamine intolerance in menopause by promoting histamine release and impairing its breakdown. A decrease in progesterone further contributes to these heightened symptoms due to its role in regulating histamine. Limited research in this area makes this a real challenge to investigate, but I include some further resources in the references on the link between estrogen, menopause and histamine intolerance. (15, 16)

Understanding the complex relationship between hormones and histamine is key, and working with a histamine-literate practitioner is a must. Now, let's shift our focus to another critical topic that's had a LOT of attention recently: the impact of viral illness on health and well-being, and how it intersects with our understanding of histamine intolerance.

Long Covid

Over the past few years, I've received a lot of messages, DMs and emails from people who've contracted Covid and then suffered from histamine intolerance and significant health issues afterwards. You, too, may have bought this book because you're suffering from Long Covid.

Early research shows that there is a link. As the world continued to fight against this virus, I dug deeper.

Histamine triggers an immune response to help fend off infections and viruses – like Covid. Studies which have investigated the link specifically between histamine, the immune system and Long Covid have demonstrated that Long Covid can activate the mast cells that release histamine (17). Research published by the International Journal of Infectious Diseases has also demonstrated that Covid hyper-inflammation and post-Covid illness may be rooted in mast cell activation syndrome (MCAS) (18). This drives up inflammation, which may cause Long Covid symptoms.

It seems that post-Covid, histamine levels may be elevated, which becomes damaging in some people. The body can respond in unpleasant ways and can cause anything from headaches to life-threatening inflammation and disease.

So what can you do about this?

Clearly, beyond what you've learned in this book, you need a sympathetic practitioner and/or doctor, depending on the severity of your symptoms. As we have acknowledged throughout, histamine issues are so individual there is no one-size-fits-all approach. You can certainly start straight away with the program in Part 2: *The Road To Recovery* and improve your diet, stress and sleep, but if you are suffering from significant post-Covid problems, you need expert help.

I recommend finding a functional medicine practitioner who has specific knowledge and experience in dealing with both histamine intolerance and Long Covid – which can be a challenge. In Chapter 7: *Low-Histamine Advanced*, I'll look at finding a good practitioner in more detail.

Practitioner or Not: That is the Question

It may seem frustrating that the recommendation is so often to "see a practitioner". It is to me as well. I'm well aware that it can sometimes feel like hitting a financial roadblock, and not everyone has the luxury of being able to afford a specialist.

As I said, I'm a journalist. I'm not a doctor (and don't want to be). However, I understand empowerment and self-education are often the best first steps in managing complex health issues like histamine intolerance, especially when professionals are just out of reach or budget.

But ultimately, finding a practitioner does help. Yes, it can be challenging on the pocket, but having someone who "gets it" is invaluable. Doing this all on your own, however much expertise you accrue, takes a lot of work. In Chapter 7: *Low-Histamine Advanced,* I'll cover this in more depth, but for now, let's arm ourselves with knowledge, insights and practical steps.

PART 2:

THE ROAD TO RECOVERY

4. Low-Histamine Diet

"The food you eat can be either the safest and most powerful form of medicine or the slowest form of poison."

– Ann Wigmore

When I was 18, I was lucky enough to travel to Italy and live there for seven months. It was a dream to escape the harsh British winter and explore such an exotic and rich culture, although admittedly, the culture I was most interested in was the calcio (soccer) and my beloved Fiorentina FC.

Having always been at the bottom of the class at school, I surprised myself by becoming almost fluent in Italian after two months. Sure, my conversations with my new friends in the Italian language were mostly calcio-related, but I was immersing myself in Italian, and I adored it. I bought *La Gazzetta dello Sport* – a pink sports newspaper – every day and devoured it sitting in the sunshine, further improving my Italian reading skills and useless soccer knowledge. I was officially an Italian soccer bore.

But I also wonder if the time I spent in Italy was the start of my histamine troubles. Being an excitable and naive 18-year-old away from home for the first time, my diet game wasn't as on point as it could have been.

I ate pizza and drank alcohol. That's pretty much it.

Every day.

Pizza washed down with alcohol. Okay, occasionally, a starter of pasta appeared before the pizzas, but it was mainly pepperoni pizza and beer (or prosecco if I found some spare change down the back of the sofa). This was the first time I can remember having stomach problems. Did this very high-histamine diet tip my body over the edge and start longer-term health issues?

Analysis of Tony's Italian "pizza" diet

- **Tomato** – high in histamine.
- **Pepperoni** – cured meat is very high in histamine. Plus, it is often pre-cooked, therefore sitting around for ages, gathering extra histamine.
- **Cheese** – it depends on the cheese, but many are high in histamine. (Mozzarella, however, is tolerated well by many.)
- **Alcohol** – sorry to break the bad news, but alcohol is one of the highest histamine things you can consume. The 18-year-old me drank a lot of Italian beer, prosecco, and grappa (a crazy Italian spirit - needless to say high histamine)
- **Gluten** – not necessarily high-histamine but potentially inflammatory (many experts caution to avoid gluten with histamine issues).

I would wash it all down with a nice, healthy chocolate (yes, high-histamine) gelato before stumbling home to my damp-smelling flat (um, hello, mold?). And by the time I left Italy, my stomach was in a mess.

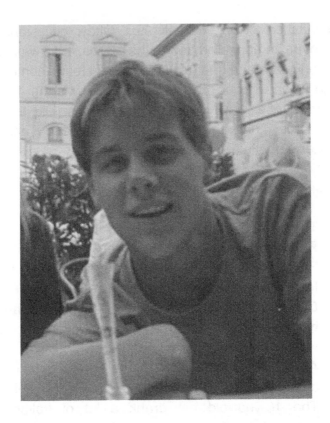

On the pizza and prosecco diet. Me in Piazza Della Repubblica, Florence at 18.

In the following years, some other issues developed – mostly gut and inflammation-related – and no doubt not helped because I drank enthusiastically on lights out. For some people, alcoholic drinks act as a potent trigger for histamine intolerance. I learned the hard way, drinking hard like most of my British friends. I settled into university where my previously refined pizza and prosecco evenings gave way to nights of beer washed down with a late-night kebab.

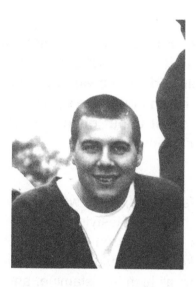

On the beer and kebab diet. Me at university at 21.

My health suffered. I became bloated and inflamed. And I could never quite work out why I would go out for some drinks with my friends, then, the next day, they were in tip-top form, while I felt like death warmed up.

(Side note: these days, I see this "early warning system" as a sort of blessing. Over the years, these histamine issues have caused me problems, but now it keeps me healthier and away from alcohol, because I know the consequences.)

Embarking on a low-histamine path can seem like you're waving goodbye to all your favorite foods. You may be thinking, "Red flag – I can see what's coming here. He's going to tell me to give up pizza, cheese, alcohol, chocolate and all the good things in life.

> **Don't worry! For every high-histamine favorite I'm encouraging you to set aside, I've got a pretty good histamine-friendly swap lined up. Admittedly, some of them aren't quite the same, but they mostly work well. It's not about giving up, it's just smart swapping for a few weeks.**

Fast forward a few years, and I was starting to live a more conventionally "healthy" lifestyle. The 30-something Tony thought he was eating an on-point diet. Pizzas were out, and avocados, kombucha and dark chocolate were in. But, surprise, they are all high in histamine, and I just ended up feeling worse and worse. Was or is that you too? If so, you are in the right place.

A 30-Day Low-Histamine Diet

This part of the book comprises four chapters,

- Low-Histamine Diet
- Low-Histamine Mindset
- Low-Histamine Lifestyle
- Low-Histamine Advanced

I suggest you implement this suggested program of changes over the course of 30 days, and see how you feel afterwards. Of course, as previously emphasized, run any changes past your doctor first, and a quick reminder, this guide is meant for information only and is no substitute for medical assistance.

As we start, I'll make some suggestions for an Easy Low-Histamine Diet. It simply means cutting out the main no-nos. Then you can see if you feel better. If this makes a difference (and it immediately worked for me), then you have some good information about histamine intolerance. You can consult Chapter 8: *Ingredient List* to learn more about specific foods.

The confusing world of histamine and food.

Some foods are low in histamine, and others are histamine-lowering. There are other foods that are high in histamine and another category of foods that are histamine-releasing (or "histamine liberators", like the tomatoes I already mentioned). Sometimes, foods can be low-histamine if they are unripe and high-histamine if they are ripe, old, or already cooked. And then sometimes the top pros totally disagree on whether something is low, medium, or high histamine.

This brings to mind the head-exploding emoji. Rest assured, in this book, I'll make it as simple as possible, with a set of rules and lists to follow that make it as easy as can be.

High histamine levels in food tend to be because of; bacteria and yeast, enzymatic activity, food processing and storage conditions, or non-microbial factors. A lot of this can get quite technical, so I'm going to make it totally straightforward, and tell you the high-histamine foods and histamine-liberating foods you want to limit over the next 30 days.

Chocolate

Listen, it's not forever, okay? I can now tolerate small amounts of chocolate. This diet is just for 30 days to see if you get better.

People with histamine intolerance are often advised to avoid chocolate. This also applies to chocolate drinks, mousses, sauces, etc. In its raw form, cacao may be less of a concern regarding histamine; however, the reason for this difference between cacao and chocolate is not entirely clear.

Try instead:

White chocolate is thought to be lower in histamine, and it suits many of my followers better. I still find I can slightly react to it, but I love white chocolate. Note: it tends to be considerably higher in sugar, which isn't good for your general health.

Carob is also relatively high in histamine, but some can stomach it just fine. Personally, it makes my knees hurt (specific, I know!)

All of this emphasizes my repeated point: tolerance to histamine-containing foods can vary from person to person, and the only way to determine your tolerance level is through self-testing. (Despite this, I guarantee there will be at least one one-star review of this book, which says: HE SAID WE CAN EAT CAROB; HE DOESN'T KNOW ANYTHING!)

One more point on chocolate. I've spent years attending some of the world's best health conferences, summits and festivals worldwide. Wherever I've gone, and whenever I've been given chocolate-based treats, it's always been accepted that chocolate with a higher cacao content and lower sugar content is better for us. That's not the case for us – and it took me a long time and many supposedly "healthy treats" to work this out.

With histamine intolerance, some 99% dark chocolate made with beautiful organic cacao beans may make you feel worse than a sugar-filled, basic milk chocolate bar bought in your local store. You may not want to rush out and buy an entire store's supply of Dairy Milk – because the sugar-filled bar isn't actually good for you. But it may just be lower in histamine or histamine-releasing properties than the rich, dark chocolate, and therefore, it will give you less of an immediate symptom flare-up.

Finally, go carefully with the low-sugar "keto chocolates" you find in health stores. These often contain inulin, xylitol, erythritol or other natural sweeteners, which may cause even more of a reaction than straight chocolate. If you have a sweet tooth, take a look at some of the satisfying recipes at the back of the book.

Fish

I can't tell you how many cans of tuna I ate as a student. Every night, me and my mates would "cook", which basically involved tipping a full can of tuna into a sachet of dried "pasta n' cheese sauce". Yum! I wonder if that played a role in my histamine intolerance.

Fish, shellfish, and other seafood products tend to contain high levels of histamine. If the fish is caught and frozen immediately, that can mean histamine levels might be lower. But you'll find most fish appear on high-histamine lists. So, mostly, fish and histamine don't go together and are unhappy bedfellows. Canned fish would fit that category.

Try instead:

Find a company that freezes the fish at sea. I use an outstanding UK company called *SeaFresh*. They freeze at sea and even have a histamine-friendly label for suitable products on their website (how many other companies do that?)

Protein-wise, while fish is often out, most fresh, organic, pasture-raised meats seem to be okay as long as they are not aged.

Leftovers

That slice of pizza still in its box from the night before? Hands off…

I used to enjoy preparing many healthy meals in advance and leaving them in the fridge. However, for the next 30 days, this is out. The longer they've been left, the more the leftovers increase in bacteria and histamine.

Try instead:

A simple solution is to freeze leftovers immediately after cooking. This means the histamine content can't then increase . Defrost thoroughly before heating them for consumption, following safety guidelines, and you'll have a freezer full of fresh low-histamine meals ready to go.

Remember, when it comes to histamine intolerance, the freezer is your friend.

Fermented foods

Fermented foods generally have higher levels of histamine as they are created using bacteria and yeast, which often increases histamine levels. Examples of fermented foods include yogurt (sad face), kombucha (you thought you were being healthy, didn't you?), sauerkraut (did you ever enjoy eating that in the first place?), and kefir (yummy, but it has to go).

Try instead:

You can make your own low-histamine yogurt. I've made a few batches of this. Two were great, one was so-so, and one... well, let's not talk about that last batch.

I make it in a pressure cooker (*Instant Pot*) on the "yogurt" setting. Heat up some coconut cream and coconut milk (or use dairy if you tolerate that) and then follow *Instant Pot* advice on making yogurt, mixing in histamine-friendly probiotics as your starter culture. (Opening up two capsules of Probiota Histaminx by Seeking Health seems to do the trick for me).

It cooks for a long time, sets in the fridge, and you're officially a yogurt maker. Who would have thought it?

Advance warning: I will not be held responsible for any fermenting mistakes you make. My most recent batch was the stuff of nightmares!

Extra note: the Instant Pot is excellent for anyone with histamine intolerance. It is a healthy, quick pressure cooker that allows you to cook low-histamine dishes. It cooks, steams, sautés, and, yes, makes histamine-intolerance-friendly yogurts. You'll find more in my other book on histamine intolerance, The Histamine Intolerance Cookbook.

Avocados

Avocados, you are joking, right? I had always presumed that avocado was the healthiest food I could eat. I bought them in bulk. High in good fats, low in carbs: the perfect food, right? But not if you're histamine intolerant. Unfair, isn't it?

Try instead:

Some good low-histamine texture swaps are pumpkin and butternut squash. Admittedly, these are a poor substitute for a lovely creamy avocado. If you must eat them, try the less-ripe green ones, as they are thought to be lower in histamine, not the very dark ones, which are super-squidgy.

Citrus

"Ugh, he banned citrus?" Well, I am not using the word "banned'" anywhere because the mysterious ways in which histamine operates mean that some people might tolerate it fine. But most histamine-intolerant-people do struggle with citrus. However, keeping it positive, don't worry. There are still plenty of ways to substitute citrus in cooking.

Try instead:

For cooking, try Verjuice. Yes, this sounds weird, and you may not have heard of it before, but it's standard in some parts of the world. It's unripe grape juice from wine regions and works excellently to replace citrus and vinegar in cooking.

Regarding replacement fruits, many histamine-friendly fruits are on the shopping list at the back of the book. My fridge is never without apples and blueberries, and indeed the blueberry made it to the front cover of this book. I also love to keep a supply of chopped frozen mango in the freezer.

Once the 30 days are up, remember to test carefully if you want to use citrus and see what works for you.

Tomato

Tomatoes are often annoyingly high in histamine. They are also histamine liberators (so they encourage the body to release histamine). This means we want to limit them and get creative in the kitchen.

Try instead:

Hands up, who misses a good old indulgent tomato pasta sauce? (Puts his own hand up.) Well, I've been working on the perfect "nomato" sauce recipe.

It contains no tomato but plenty of carrot, onion, pumpkin, sweet potato and beetroot. It's coming later in the book.

FAQ: What's the difference between histamine-containing foods and histamine liberators?

Histamine-containing foods naturally have histamine in them. This includes things like aged cheeses, most fish, and avocados.

Histamine liberators, on the other hand, don't contain histamine but create conditions for it to be produced in the body. They encourage your body to release its own histamine. Foods like citrus fruits, tomatoes, and chocolate are histamine liberators. And some foods are both high-histamine and histamine liberators.

Cheeses

Many kinds of cheese are like a histamine bomb in your tummy—especially the blue, veiny ones. So you're cutting most of them out for the next 30 days.

Just remember, this is not a permanent thing. The goal is to lower those histamine levels and then slowly bring back some of your favorite cheesy treats while paying attention to what your body can handle.

Try instead:

No one wants to miss out on a good cheese platter. Stick to softer cheeses such as mozzarella and ricotta. These suit many people with histamine intolerance (including me), but not everybody, so test them with caution. There's a complete list of cheeses at the back of this book, but as a rule, hard cheeses = higher in histamine.

Alcohol

Alcohol tends to be very high in histamine. Red wine and its fancy friends, like prosecco, seem to be some of the worst culprits. So, watch out for those.

Try instead:

For the first 30 days, ideally, you'll cut out all alcohol. But if you're craving a drink and you really can't do without, some types of alcohol seem to be (a bit) more histamine-friendly.

Members of the histamine community have shared their experiences of enjoying a drink while minimizing adverse effects. It's not about heavy drinking, but savoring a glass or two.

Tequila gets a lot of love. On the very rare occasion when I drink these days I might choose it. Elsewhere, a particular clean vodka called Tito's seems to suit people a little better than others. This is easier to find in the USA.

You could also try the various "wine wands" out there. I tried a bestseller called The Wand. It has 9,399 positive ratings at an average of 4.2 (at the time of writing).

It is described as a "Histamine and Sulfite Filter, Purifier Alleviates Wine Allergies & Headaches, Stir Stick Aerates Wine," so you can imagine how excited I was at being able to tolerate wine again.

I tested it with a glass of wine I was planning to use for cooking. Unfortunately, I had a bit of a reaction. I was wearing an Oura Ring on my thumb, which tracks my heart rate, and it was elevated after drinking the filtered red wine. But it may work better for you. I haven't used it since and have given up on red wine, but I'm open to being persuaded again.

Should I be talking about which alcohol to drink in a book dedicated to health and histamine? I believe so. My goal is to help you make lasting changes, and many people reading this don't want to give up everything good in life entirely – especially alcohol.

Ideally, you should restrict alcohol when following a low-histamine diet. If you really can't bear to do that, then follow the above suggestions with as much moderation as possible. Of course, as always, be mindful of your drinking.

To summarize, there is a wide range of foods that individuals with histamine intolerance or sensitivities are commonly advised to monitor or avoid. Here is a list of many of the foods to watch, while acknowledging that everybody is different, and tolerance levels vary wildly. Remember, this is not forever. It is for the next month, to see how you feel afterwards.

- Aged cheese and hard cheese
- Alcohol (red wine, I'm looking at you!)
- Avocado
- Bananas
- Beans and pulses
- Chocolate (especially very dark chocolate)
- Citrus fruits (most)
- Coffee (maybe – this is a much debated area. More in Chapter 7: *Low-Histamine Advanced*)
- Cured meats
- Dried fruits (though some people are okay with these)
- Eggs, (opinion very split – read more below in the Low-Histamine Shopping List section)
- Energy drinks

- Fermented foods
- Foods with vinegar (though Apple Cider Vinegar might be okay)
- Leftovers, unless frozen immediately
- Nuts (though some lists suggest certain nuts are okay)
- Papaya
- Pineapple
- Pickled or canned foods
- Shellfish
- Smoked fish (stick to fresh from the water or the freezer)
- Soy products
- Soured foods
- Spinach
- Strawberries
- Tea
- Tomatoes
- Most artificial preservatives

So, what can I eat over the next 30 days?

Basically, everything else. It is actually a very healthy and tasty diet, and you'll enjoy some delicious new combinations.

There is a complete shopping list at the back of the book. But here is a list of some of my favorite low-histamine foods that I stock my kitchen with.

As always, test carefully.

Low-histamine Shopping List

These are foods that tend to be lower in histamine. Note: everybody is different. Some are far more sensitive, and some far less. This is a partial list; there is a complete ingredient list in the Low-Histamine Survival Kit section at the back of the book.

- Fresh meat: beef, chicken, turkey, lamb, pork and most other meats. Organic is best, but it is far more expensive, unfortunately. Avoid aged meat (this is important). Freeze if you like, for extra freshness.
- Fresh fruit: blueberries, apples, mangoes, peaches, grapes, and pears are some of my faves. I love eating frozen fruit as a treat – particularly blueberries and mango.
- Frozen fish: frozen at sea – use a company like SeaFresh (who only operate in the UK unfortunately). Or catch it yourself and cook it on the boat!
- Eggs: 0pinion is split on eggs. They were initially thought to be a histamine liberator, and when I've run polls on the site, some of my followers avoid them. But not all. Thankfully, I can tolerate them, but test very carefully.
- Fresh veggies: the list is long; celery, arugula, radishes, lettuce, potato, sweet potato, broccoli, cauliflower, cabbage, pea shoots, carrots, zucchini and cucumbers are some of my faves). I include onions, which are said to include anti-histamine properties. Check individual veggies in the food list at the back of the book and avoid spinach.
- The softer cheeses: as I emphasized previously, softer cheeses like ricotta and mozzarella tend to be tolerated well by most.
- Grains and starches: rice, oats, quinoa, corn and potatoes.
- Other bits: flaxseed (ground and sprouted if possible), rice, extra virgin olive oil, juices, coconut milk)
- Herbs: basil, thyme, turmeric, and lots more; check the complete list in the Low-Histamine Survival Kit section

One of the interesting things about histamine intolerance and diet is you never really know about any individual food. Indeed, you might be surprised at some of the foods I've included here. That's because we are all different, and that's why (IMHO) this book is so necessary.

If you need more clarification about a particular food, I would direct you to a resource in the Low-Histamine Survival Kit section called Food Polls. To get more information on some of these seemingly random and contradictory medium foods, I've been crowdsourcing knowledge for several years through a series of food polls on my Instagram. The results are often fascinating. These are obviously entirely non-scientific and certainly not double-blind placebo-controlled studies. It's just polling a lot of people at once to get a general feel for what people tend to tolerate and what they tend not to. Allow them to guide you and consider them a small, helpful, but unscientific resource as you continue your journey on histamine intolerance.

LOWER YOUR HISTAMINE LEVELS WITH FOOD

Did you know that pea shoots are renowned for their histamine-lowering properties? That's right – consuming pea shoots can actually help reduce histamine levels in your body. They're not only nutritious but also a natural way to combat histamine. I buy them by the bucket-load (thanks, Ocado) and am also taking a tentative step towards growing them for a fresher supply. Incorporating pea shoots into your meals could be a delicious and healthful strategy in managing histamine levels.

Histamine isn't inherently bad. It's about managing your unique threshold, which varies due to factors like gut health and genetics.

Consider our hunter-gatherer ancestors, who naturally consumed lower-histamine diets. While we can't replicate their lifestyle, (er, I'm not giving up my fridge or my coffee machine) choosing unprocessed, organic foods aligns with this ancestral approach, potentially reducing histamine-related issues.

How should I expect to feel on the low-histamine diet?

Many people find that reducing histamine intake starts to quickly alleviate some of their symptoms. If you've noticed an improvement, that's fantastic. If not, don't despair; diet might not be your only trigger. We'll be looking at all sorts of other ways our histamine levels can spike in the body, and what to do about it.

In fact, in Chapter 5: *Low-Histamine Mindset*, I examine the compelling research linking histamine and stress. It's wild to think that being hunched over our laptop at 1 a.m. replying to an email from Bob in accounts might be linked to histamine intolerance. But it is (thanks, Bob). And what astonished me even more is the fact that the connection goes both ways. Histamine intolerance isn't just *caused* by stress; it's also *a cause* of it, which underlines just how pivotal our mindset is in this journey.

LOW-HISTAMINE DIET AT-A-GLANCE

- ☐ Spot and cut out high-histamine foods; embrace low-histamine alternatives
- ☐ Focus on histamine-friendly meat, veggies, fruit and other options on the low-histamine shopping list
- ☐ Use cooking methods that keep histamine to a minimum (such as pressure cookers and freezing leftovers)
- ☐ Try for 30 days and see how you feel

5. Low-Histamine Mindset

"Your body hears everything your mind says."

– Naomi Judd

Over the years, I've noticed a distinct pattern. My histamine intolerance symptoms flare up when I'm overly stressed, buried in work, or neglecting self-care. By contrast, my symptoms recede when I step back and prioritize relaxation and quality time with loved ones. Holidays are the best. My symptoms miraculously almost disappear every time.

This isn't mere coincidence. There is compelling research that shows why many of us seem to have reduced histamine symptoms when we spend less time hunched over our laptops at 1 a.m. replying to those emails from the aforementioned Bob in accounts. It ties back to our body's rest and repair powerhouse: the parasympathetic nervous system. Tapping into this system allows our body to prioritize healing, overreacting to stress. Yet, amid the challenge of managing histamine intolerance alongside everyday life, many of us struggle to access this crucial state.

What to expect in this chapter:

Coming up, I focus on finding balance by reducing stress and developing a practice of rest and reflection. We'll look at two key areas:

Histamine Healing Meditations: When dealing with histamine intolerance, adequate rest isn't a luxury—it's a necessity. We'll delve deeper into how we can repattern our behavior to ensure you're giving your body the downtime it needs to recover. (Side note: Now, if you're anything like me, you might be tempted to gloss over this part, thinking, 'Sure, mindfulness... heard it all before.' Please give it a chance. You won't heal properly without calming your body and mind.)

Histamine Healing Mindset: Reflect on your healing process and enhance your recovery. This is a crucial step in understanding your body's unique responses, enabling you to pinpoint what works best for you. By reflecting on and noting down your experiences, we can begin to craft a recovery plan just for you.

The important link between stress and histamine intolerance

The impact of histamine intolerance extends beyond physical symptoms, profoundly affecting our mental state and brain function. This can significantly impact how you feel mentally and physically, as research has found that histamine issues have all sorts of mental and brain impacts. For example, "dysfunction of the histamine system may underlie some forms of apathy" and "a potentially critical player in the pathology of depression, histamine". Numerous studies draw a clear line between histamine levels and mental well-being, yet this is the connection people often miss. (1,2,3,4,5).

So, what is the parasympathetic nervous system, and why is it important? It's the "rest-and-digest" healing response. It's the opposite of "fight-or-flight". It plays an important role in regulating our body's response to stress and anxiety. When it kicks in, it helps slow down our heart rate, decrease our blood pressure, and promote relaxation throughout the body. Sometimes it can help us slow down the heart rate and hit the reset button on all that tension and stress. (6)

Without the parasympathetic nervous system, we could not calm down after experiencing a stressful event like a histamine flare-up (which elevates our sympathetic nervous system). *Sympathetic* sounds good right? Nope. Our bodies remain in a heightened state of sensitivity, unless that parasympathetic good stuff can kick in. In the long term, your nervous system being stuck on *sympathetic* would lead to being unable to heal and lighten the bucket.

All of this means we must focus even harder on our mental approach to histamine intolerance, as the symptoms make it even harder to retain a positive outlook. On a personal note, the deep mental fog that accompanies a flare-up is not pleasant. Let's deal with that as much as we can.

Histamine Healing Meditations

"The greatest weapon against stress is our ability to choose one thought over another."

– William James

Writing about histamine intolerance has not traditionally been my day job. Normally I spend my time writing books and recording podcasts using the advanced mindset techniques of Neuro-Linguistic Programming (NLP) and energy psychology. And that's why I'm particularly excited about this part of the book. Because, as we've seen, there's a significant link to my primary work. These mindset techniques and the parasympathetic nervous system are essential for healing from histamine intolerance and dealing with the intense pressure it puts on our body and mind.

My aim is not just to make these episodes more bearable but to provide you with effective strategies to manage your mental health and heal quicker. I hope to guide you through any similar experiences and enhance your resilience when they occur.

In this part of the book, I want to ensure that the fight-or-flight response you may experience with histamine intolerance gets switched off as much as possible, and then encourage some long-term healing habits. As we now know, you can't heal until we calm your nervous system. And for inspiration, we're going to travel back in time.

In ancient Japan, there existed a practice called ūgen. It's a term that doesn't have a direct translation in English but refers to the profound grace and subtlety found in the natural world. Japanese monks would sit in nature, absorbing the serenity around them — the distant call of a bird, the whisper of wind through bamboo. They believed these moments of deep introspection had curative powers. They inherently recognized the healing benefits of quiet reflection.

In a world where modern ailments such as histamine intolerance challenge us, I've found that turning to such instinctive, natural, time-honored practices can be helpful. In other words, as counter-intuitive as it may seem, it's not too much of a leap to suggest that embracing moments of stillness as ancient Japanese monks did can help with very modern problems like histamine intolerance. You just have to give it a chance and allow it to provide a gentle, natural respite for your body and mind.

I encourage you to set aside ten minutes each day for the next 30 days to switch off and truly rest. It's really not long when you think about it. Yet, as science has already seen, this simple act might profoundly affect your histamine symptoms, more than anything else. It's been a game-changer for my symptoms, though it's not an immediate fix and requires some consistency. And don't worry, we won't be following the exact "mysterious profundity" rituals of the monks. We'll just be taking inspiration from their appreciation of quiet moments in nature.

Healing demands adequate rest.

We will be switching off and resting for these short periods during the day, using a combination of meditation and hypnosis. Much like the profound depth in yūgen, this combination takes us deep into an altered, more relaxed state, offering a transformative experience that draws from ancient wisdom and modern techniques.

Meditation has an amazing influence on your brain. It is a special tool that offers a lot of benefits in the fight against histamine intolerance (although, of course, it's not a magic pill). Benefits like:

- A bolstered immune system – think of it as your body's very own in-built defense upgrade (which is crucial when your body is fighting histamine overload)
- A tangible decrease in stress, anxiety, and depression – meditation can transform your mind into a more

    peaceful, manageable space (which is vital with hista-
    mine issues, as we've seen)
- Improved sleep quality – essential for repairing and
  rejuvenating your body amid histamine challenges.

Then, we combine that with hypnosis, which can reprogram your mind to tackle stress and recharge. This is particularly important when fighting histamine intolerance's debilitating effects. Hypnosis is effective at treating anxiety (7), improving deep sleep and insomnia (8), and improving symptoms of fatigue (9).

I offer two Histamine Healing Meditations combining hypnosis, meditation and setting intentions around histamine intolerance below. But really, you can use any meditation or hypnosis technique, app, download or process. It's just a question of allowing your body and mind to catch up with some long-awaited downtime.

Histamine Healing Meditation 1

"There's a reason that they call it a practice. It's not a magic pill. It's something you have to do. But the more you do it, the more you see results."

– Dan Harris

Inspired by Betty Erickson, one of my favorite hypnosis and meditation teachers, this trance session has been a go-to for my clients and me for many years. I've gently adapted it here specifically for histamine intolerance. If you practice this outdoors, you'll notice a pleasing resonance with the concept of yūgen we explored earlier.

- Be still. Set an intention for the next ten minutes. How would you like to feel about your histamine intolerance after the ten minutes is up?
- Concentrate on three things you can see. Go slowly, letting your gaze linger on each, in an unrushed manner..
- Now, put your attention on three things you can hear. Again, there is no rush; allow each sound its moment.
- You can now focus on three things you can feel or touch. Let each sensation unfurl at its own pace.
- Continue this sensory circuit, methodically cycling through sights, sounds, and sensations. Try to vary your picks each time. These can be anything external that your senses tune into: people, items, objects, nature, and so on.

As you cycle through these sights, sounds, and sensations, you'll probably notice the gently hypnotic resonance in bringing all your attention to your senses. Remember, the more you commit to doing this daily, the more you'll notice the benefits.

Histamine Healing Meditation 2

Dive deep into the history of hypnotherapy, and you'll uncover a subtle and transformative gem: the Reverse Counting Technique. The pioneers of hypnosis recognized the power of numerical sequences in diverting the conscious mind. They found the act of counting, especially backwards and starting from an unusually high number, became a cognitive task that required complete focus.

It's challenging for the mind to hold onto worries about something like histamine intolerance when it's juggling numbers in reverse. By the time you're several numbers down, you've not only interrupted your usual thought process but effectively created a mental detour, ushering in a state of relaxation.

So again, this hypnotic exercise hinges on channeling your mind's full attention to a single activity. The better you get at this, the more your concerns begin to dissolve, for the mind can't juggle this focus and worry concurrently.

- Be still. Set an intention for this ten-minute meditation. How would you like to feel about your histamine intolerance after the ten minutes is up?
- At a stressful moment, take deep breaths and count backward from the number 100,000 for one minute, like this: 100,000, 99,999, 99,998, 99,997. If you lose your place or get the numbers wrong, return to 100,000 and start again.
- Do this for ten minutes. By wholly occupying your conscious mind, you start to quiet all the (often unhelpful) internal chatter around histamine intolerance. At the end, if you're like me, you may want to sit quietly for a while and *not* count anymore!

The more challenging you find this, the more likely it is that you need it. It is tricky to concentrate on the numbers and get them right. This is good – the change in where you are directing your attention is important.

Remember, you can try these hypnotic techniques as a starting point. I present them here because that's my area of specialty, but honestly, I'd be thrilled if you do any form of meditation, hypnosis, trance, rest, prayer, silence, sleep, or other downtime activity that allows your mind to rest and your body to heal.

Histamine Healing Meditation 3

Over the years, lots of people have said versions of this to me;

"But Tony, finding rest is challenging for me. Meditation isn't my thing, and I'm not the type to gaze at candles."

I get it. Sitting quietly for ten minutes and counting or noticing stuff isn't for everyone. Your third option (the one most of my clients go for and love) is to try guided hypnosis meditations. I'd love to encourage you to try my meditation and hypnosis programs, and you can find loads of specific healing resources of mine on my program called The Healthy AF Method – www.tonywrighton.com/healthy.

The beauty of The Healthy AF Method is that my students don't require any candle-staring or fancy yoga positions. They just find a quiet moment in their day, pop in their headphones, and let my guided session do the rest. Consider it an invest-ment in yourself, a wellness tool designed for real people living in a real, hectic world – with no mystical fluff.

I've even recorded a very specific Histamine Healing Medita-tion which you can listen to every day.

Remember, if you struggle to unwind and relax, you may exacerbate your histamine symptoms, for all the reasons we've already outlined. You want to create an environment in your body and mind where you can start to heal.

Histamine Healing Mindset

"What's measured, improves."

– Peter Drucker

Here are some questions for you around histamine intolerance.

- How do you react when you eat eggs? Do you feel better or worse?
- Do you react to nuts? Specifically, which nuts? For example, cashews may make you feel worse, while almonds are fine.
- Do magnesium supplements help your histamine Intolerance symptoms?
- Does taking a hot bath make you feel better or worse?
- When you meditate, do you think your symptoms decrease?

Remember, what's measured improves, and when you don't collect any metrics, you will often just be guessing at what works. It may not seem sexy to check your data or fill in a spreadsheet before you go to bed at night, but it can be. Um, well, I think it is.

Now we're going to craft our very own tailored low-histamine approach by tracking sleep, diet, health, and workouts and even diving into advanced insights like HRV (Heart Rate Variability) and genetic markers from DNA. You ask yourself: what works best? And then you know you should keep doing it. By monitoring your progress and responses, you will refine your strategy and cultivate a proactive mindset, empowering you to take control of your histamine journey.

This movement is known as Quantified Self; it involves collecting data to achieve "self-knowledge through numbers". We are all different, so I encourage you to track all your symptoms, diet and activities for yourself and see what's working best.

These stats will be the basis for your personal histamine intolerance template.

How The Histamine Intolerance Symptom Tracker Works

Each evening, I encourage you to turn to the back of the book and fill out the Histamine Intolerance Symptom Tracker I've included there. From those questions, we'll start to decipher which foods make you feel better, which ones make you feel low, what gives you energy, improves your mood, and gives you a boost and which parts of the program in this book have worked well, or not so well.

Then, anytime you need more clarification about a food, practice, or something you've changed, you can analyze your tracking metrics.

You'll find my basic Histamine Intolerance Symptom Tracker in the Low-Histamine Survival Kit. But you can follow your own preferred way of collecting metrics. For example, I have been doing this for so long that I fill out a Google spreadsheet; it is the quickest way, and offers a little more detail. The nightly process takes less than 30 seconds, and then the spreadsheet is there for me to study when needed.

> **If you are interested in using apps, try Symple and Symptom Tracker+, or you could even try MyFitnessPal. The key is finding a reliable way to spot potentially significant trends in your data – I now have years' worth of data to go and check.**

Next time you try to figure out if something has been effective, you will have the data there to prove what works. You will have collected your own energy evidence—Bye-bye guesswork.

- Dedicate two minutes every evening to recording your metrics.
- Use the 30-day grid at the back of this book to jot down symptoms and reflections.
- Review the data periodically to identify patterns and effective strategies. For instance, if exercising consistently reduces your symptoms, take note.
- Arm yourself with insights for the future. Trust in the data – over time, it will be a valuable guide.
- Embrace a proactive mindset, continually assessing and adapting based on your findings to optimize your well-being.

WHAT METRICS TO COLLECT: THE PAPAYA MIGHT HAVE TO GO

You can collect data points on sleep, diet, heart health, exercise and just about anything else you can think of. So, what should you collect metrics on?

I encourage you to get creative. I've put basic options in the Histamine Intolerance Symptom Tracker at the back of the book, but there's a notes section where you can jot down just about anything. Use that liberally.

For instance, if you suspect a significant increase in symptoms every time you eat papaya, you might want to track your papaya consumption (reminder: papaya is generally considered high in histamine; it is kryptonite for me). If the metrics prove a link between papaya and feeling low, you can then decide whether the papaya will have to go. We aim for a level of personalized detail that will reveal hidden but important revelations about your personal histamine reactions.

Potential areas to track

- Symptom severity
- Foods you aren't sure about
- Amount of food
- Time of meals
- Drink (especially alcohol)
- Energy
- Mood
- Focus
- Workout length and quality
- Length of sleep
- Quality of sleep
- What time you went to bed
- Heart rate
- Heart rate variability
- Food eaten
- Supplements taken (this is a really important one to track)

- Any of the techniques in this book
- Papaya consumption! And so on…

For the subjective areas above, such as energy or happiness levels, mark yourself with a number out of 10. You could also use a percentage.

I am an unashamed nerd when it comes to tracking stuff. It has to take less than 60 seconds at night, though, because who wants to spend hours doing this stuff? I track anything and everything— lifestyle factors, supplements, energy levels, sleep quality, and anything else I'm focusing on.

There is no limit to what you might track. Years ago, I realized I suffered from stomach problems after eating nuts. But not all nuts. So, I collected some nut metrics. (That's a sentence I never thought I'd utter in public.) A month after I'd started my unique experiment (I'm sad, I know), I'd uncovered the culprit – cashew nuts were making me bloated. This was before I learned about histamine, but now it's clear why cashews were so troublesome for me. Nowadays, I avoid what I call "the evil cashew," and my gut is much happier for it.

So, pick a few areas to track. As you go through the book, add anything that you think might be having a big positive (or negative) impact.

Symptom Tracker Tip

One of the areas we dive into on my online program The Healthy AF Method is using AI to help with symptom tracking. We use ChatGPT and other AI providers to help analyze our metrics and ask for correlations or suggestions. As weird as it may sound, the tech is improving so fast we are often surprised at what it spots. The human eye misses stuff that the AI picks up. AI is going to be so important in the future of healthcare and dealing with complex conditions like histamine intolerance. Check out www.tonywrighton.com/healthy for more.

Measuring recovery

My histamine symptoms have led to serious health issues, including a severe case of burnout when I ended up in bed for a few months. I found this system of figuring out what works in my recovery and healing journey helpful at that point and have done ever since. I tracked energy (as that was the thing I was lacking) and then some other parameters.

Only later, when I discovered the concept of histamine intolerance, did I layer in more specific histamine factors.

Over a period of years, some fascinating trends developed.

I ended up stumbling upon something strange that my spreadsheet proved time and time again:

Unplugging from screens boosted my energy by up to 20% per day.

I tracked this by completely switching off in manageable two-hour chunks and then noting it.

Clearly, this was not scientific research, but there is an increasing body of science on this. It shows that excessive tech and screen use can contribute to burnout. It overwhelms the brain, causes a state of constant stimulation, and leads to increased levels of stress and fatigue (10, 11) – not good for histamine intolerance.

"Constant exposure to devices like smartphones, personal computers, and television can severely affect mental health – increase stress and anxiety, for example, and cause various sleep issues in both children as well as adults…. Oftentimes it can cause the induction of a state of hyper-arousal, increase stress hormones, desynchronize the body clock or the circadian cycle, alter brain chemistry and create a drag on mental energy and development."

Increased Screen Time as a Cause of Declining Physical, Psychological Health, and Sleep Patterns – Vaishnavi S Nakshine et al

---

Exploring Tech Aids for Symptom Tracking

As well as all the free tracking options outlined above, what about the wide range of smart watches, rings, bands and other health tech out there? I like tracking rings like Oura Ring and Ultrahuman. They fit snugly on your finger and Oura gained attention for its ability to detect Covid-19 symptoms three days in advance. (12)

> These trackers don't provide direct insights into histamine intolerance, but can offer valuable insights into areas like heart rate and Heart Rate Variability (HRV). It's useful for monitoring overall well-being, and certainly a lower resting heart rate and higher HRV are generally positive indicators (though this isn't medical advice). For me, these rings are a nice extra tool to track health parameters.

Another interesting thing I've learned from tracking is that a workout increases my energy levels by an average of 5.4% per day.

The more exercise I do, the better I feel. It just seems to help. And it doesn't have to be strenuous exercise, either. It could be anything from a long walk to a gym workout or playing tennis with my buddies. These different forms of exercise help me feel good and energized.

Again, it's not a double-blind, placebo-controlled study, but it's good enough for me. These relaxed forms of exercise are the opposite of stress, which seems to help lower my histamine bucket.

I wanted to mention exercise briefly as some people find their histamine levels increase with strenuous workouts. These people may have to focus less on grunt-inducing heavy weights and more on calming forms of exercise like yoga, Qi Gong or walking. Sometimes this will have to be extremely gentle. (Obviously, liaise with your practitioner). Then, when their symptoms die down, and their histamine levels are reduced, they can hopefully return to more regular levels of exercise. I cover this in detail in Chapter 7: *Low-Histamine Advanced*.

Next, we'll look at more lifestyle changes that can rapidly decrease your histamine levels and significantly enhance your wellbeing.

LOW-HISTAMINE MINDSET AT-A-GLANCE

- ☐ **Understand Stress: learn how continuous stress worsens histamine symptoms**
- ☐ **Unlock Calm: hypnosis and meditation can be game-changers in your histamine intolerance journey**
- ☐ **Use "Histamine Healing Meditations": shift from over-stimulation to a healing state**
- ☐ **Use the Histamine Intolerance Symptom Tracker: Monitor your progress and figure out what works**

6. Low-Histamine Lifestyle

"You can't control everything in your life, but you can control your lifestyle."

– Mandy Ingber

My university days. Ah, the memories. It was a time of too much beer, caffeine and housing that, let's be honest, was more budget-friendly than health-friendly. I was living in Leamington Spa in England, and my rent was £26 a week (about $30). That got me the kind of student digs you might imagine: a place with character, but not always the good kind. I had a lot of problems with inflammation at that time, but I chalked them up to late nights, student diet, and a love of kebabs with garlic sauce at 2 a.m. Maybe I should have been looking at the damp patches on the ceiling instead…

As I've mentioned, I also lived for a time in Florence, Italy. I was living right in the midst of history in Santo Spirito, immersed in Italian culture, with every bit of that old-world charm. But that charm came with a unique musty scent every time I entered my flat. Ancient buildings are beautiful until you realize you're probably not the only living thing in there. My health worsened. Was it really the non-stop pizza or was there something in the walls?

It took me some time (and, admittedly, a bit of denial) to join the dots. Perhaps I should have known. You've already seen that picture of "Inflamed Tony" at university…

The spaces we occupy and the lifestyle we lead often play a surprisingly important role in managing our histamine intolerance symptoms. Factors such as the air we breathe, the conditions of our living or working spaces, electromagnetic fields, and even seemingly minor details like moisture and humidity can affect our body's histamine levels. So in this chapter, we will consider our environment. We'll also examine whether supplements or medication can help us on our low-histamine journey. But I start with an area that stands out as a prevalent and potentially harmful environmental factor when it comes to histamine intolerance. In fact, it's the very reason I ended up writing this book in the first place, but it took me an extraordinarily long time to realize it.

Mold

Long-term mold exposure is considered one of the leading causes of histamine intolerance, and I promised earlier that we'd look at this in more detail. Is it possible you are suffering from past or present mold exposure, which is contributing to or causing your histamine intolerance?

Let's explore how you can ensure your surroundings contribute to your health rather than undermine it. The most pressing matter is to check your environment for mold.

Mold can hide behind walls, floors, ceilings and chimneys. Sometimes mold is very obvious, and sometimes it's hiding somewhere but still causing problems.

You could start with a pinless moisture meter on the walls to determine if you live in a damp home, but this is a limited solution that only goes so far. If you find moisture or mold, this is good information, but don't try cleaning the mold yourself.

This is a common mistake that may release spores into the environment and make you feel even worse.

The gold standard is calling in comprehensive experts to check for mold. For instance, Building Forensics is a very reputable company in the UK and highly respected. They will come to your house and follow these steps:

- Assessing symptoms, reaction history and medical prognosis (if available).
- Visual and olfactory survey to assess construction and design defects.
- Particle counts to determine high risk hyphal fragments.
- Specific and humidity ratios (function of RH and temperature) to evaluate risk areas.
- Thermal imaging to risk assess target areas.
- Moisture mapping of risk areas identified.
- Various forms of sampling and lab analysis, depending on budget or need.

The process is in-depth and technical; if you live in a mold-affected house, it may be a necessary investment. But, unfortunately, it is not cheap. This is a considerable investment that, price-wise, is only available to some.

Remember that ongoing mold exposure issues can sometimes be caused by an environment that isn't your house, such as your office or somewhere you visit regularly. For example, I was previously a member of a rather lovely gym in West London that I ended up never going to again.

Why? Every time I went to work out, I'd feel great afterwards. So far, so good. But the next day, I'd always feel anxious and ungrounded, and sometimes have stomach issues. Because this reaction was delayed by 24 hours, it unfortunately took me a long time to figure out.

But eventually, I did – it was something to do with the air quality.

This gym was located in a basement, so there were probably air quality or mold issues. When I inspected more closely, I saw a small but significant amount of mold on the walls in the showers too, which would also do it.

Now I go to a gym with windows.

In addition, you might be living in a nice, warm, non-moldy house now but have suffered previous exposure (remember my student digs?). That would mean you might still be getting symptoms, even if you've now escaped the moldy environment. You will want to find a good test to help you assess if your symptoms are partly down to mold exposure, past or present.

The Great Plains Mycotoxin test is a good one that may be helpful. This is the one that helped explain so much for me. You'll also want a practitioner to help you assess the results (more on this in Chapter 7: *Low-Histamine Advanced*), as, without a specialist to guide you, it isn't obvious what to do next.

Air quality

All of the above means air quality is particularly important to me and many people with histamine issues. It has been particularly top of mind since I did that Great Plains Mycotoxins test, which revealed that I have significant levels of mycotoxins.

This means previous black mold exposure is almost certainly the reason behind my own histamine intolerance.

It means I'm now conscientious about air quality and sensitive to mold; if you are histamine intolerant, you are probably sensitive to mold too.

Most of us think that air pollution is something that happens outside; 90% of our time is, on average, spent indoors. The air we breathe inside is often even worse. It can be up to five times more polluted with mold, chemical gases, carpet fibers, dust, bacteria, viruses, pollution and toxins from overcooked food (a big one).

DO I REALLY NEED TO WORRY ABOUT AIR QUALITY?

The World Health Organization (WHO) has listed air quality as the single biggest environmental threat to public health. The air we breathe is directly linked to our health. Poor air quality is consistently linked to a laundry list of health complaints (13), including histamine intolerance (14).

So, how do we clean the air in our homes? Here are two options. Neither option will cure your histamine intolerance or mold issues, but they will help to lessen your symptoms if they are environmentally-based.

1. Costly option: get a state-of-the-art air purifier.
2. Free option: use the German tradition of *luften*. Luften is a word for the German national obsession with room ventilation. It is such a part of the national fabric

that luften is regularly observed in schools and homes – basically, opening a window to let in some fresh air. This can be chilly in winter but generally means better indoor air. Remember, it does not stop pollution from coming in from outside if you live near road traffic.

A deep dive on air purifiers

You want a purifier that – as far as possible – gets rid of mold spores and allergens like pollen, dust, dust mite feces (ugh), and pet dander (which is especially important if you have pets).

Then you also want them to get rid of Chemicals and Volatile Organic Compounds (VOCs), bacteria, viruses and triggering smells. You want one with a decent HEPA filter (the gold standard for filters) and one that is not too noisy – you don't want to feel like you are sleeping in an industrial plant.

I've spent far too many hours of my life down the rabbit hole trying to find the best air purifiers. I mainly use one in my bedroom, and I have noticed a difference in my overnight stuffy nose levels (another technical term). My sleep has improved considerably. The first time I used it, I felt like I'd been inhaling lovely, cool forest air all night. That meant I felt livelier the following day. I also noticed that being close to certain heaters/radiators in my house makes me feel suboptimal. It's like a heavy headache, and I can't really explain why it happens. This particularly happens in winter when the windows tend to be closed more. However, when I open a window or plug in the purifier, that headache feeling dissipates, and I breathe better.

One particularly popular air purifier brand is The Air Doctor. It comes with UltraHEPA filters. HEPA is an efficiency standard for air filters; the acronym stands for "high-efficiency particulate absorbing filter and high-efficiency particulate arrestance filter". These are 100x more effective than ordinary HEPA filters, capturing 99.99% of particles down to .003 microns. So, that's almost 100% of particles.

The Air Doctor comes with a hefty price tag of around $500, so you'll be pleased to hear that, while I do find air purifiers helpful, after much experimentation, I've decided opening a window wide works even better!

Household products

"Living a healthy lifestyle is a choice. We choose health, or we choose disease."

– Joyce Meyer

Okay, let's talk toothpaste. We are now getting into territory that anybody who doesn't suffer from histamine intolerance may regard as bonkers. That's alright, though. We're on our own path here and aware of what's at stake. There is an ingredient known as a synthetic detergent in toothpaste that causes many people to get mouth ulcers. It's called Sodium Lauryl Sulfate or SLS. If you have mouth ulcers then when you switch toothpaste, you might find that they magically go away.

That's what happened to me. I used to get mouth ulcers until I switched to natural toothpaste. Then I found out that other people in the histamine world report the same thing, and the science suggests SLS may be a contributing factor. (15) If you take away nothing else from this book, perhaps you'll stop getting mouth ulcers – that's a major win, right?

Elsewhere, it seems clear that many people with histamine intolerance are particularly sensitive to smells and certain products. Watch out for particularly intense smells and fragrances, such as certain cleaning products and air fresheners. Even nail varnish and nail varnish remover can be directly or indirectly triggering, as well as common perfumes.

For this book, I dug into the research, and, from a personal perspective, I've found it somewhat gratifying that the science shows I'm not alone in being ridiculously sensitive to how things smell.

"Perfume induces a dose-dependent non-IgE-mediated histamine release from human peripheral blood basophils. Increased basophil reactivity to perfume was found in patients with respiratory symptoms related to perfume". (16)

There are quite a few apps out there that can help in this area. Think Dirty, or EWG's Skin Deep sites are helpful, and an app called Yuka is very popular, too. Scan the products in your bathroom cabinet, and get color-coded science and research on the ingredients. You might be surprised at how many supposedly "natural" products show up as irritants or toxic. As a result of using these sites, I've changed many of the products I have around the home.

SMELLS I'M SENSITIVE TO

Here's a short list of nasty niffs I'm more sensitive to than others because of histamine issues. If this is you too, then hey, you are not alone.

- **Perfume**
- **Nail varnish**
- **Scented candles (the worst – I can smell them three rooms away)**
- **Fresh paint**
- **Cleaning products**
- **New carpet**
- **Glue**
- **Car exhaust fumes**
- **Chlorine in pools**
- **And even a newly opened marker pen**

Remember, this is not an exhaustive list, and your triggers may differ from mine.

Also, beware: "natural" is not always better. I already mentioned how we recently switched to a particularly smelly rhubarb floor cleaner in our home. This was a reputable, plant-based, eco-friendly brand. In fact on their website, it describes their rhubarb floor cleaner thus;

"...smells so good, you practically want to eat off the floor."

Er, no. I do not exaggerate when I say that this rhubarb floor cleaner was one of the most gag-inducing smells I've ever experienced, and I couldn't get rid of it for days.

Remember, the label "natural" isn't a free pass. Sometimes, even the most eco-friendly products can still kick up a histamine fuss. And as for that rhubarb floor cleaner, I'll pass on that "floor-dining" experience, thank you.

Electromagnetic Fields (EMFs)

"Whenever a patient presents with symptoms suggestive of mast cell activation syndrome, I immediately enquire about their exposures to electrical fields, magnetic fields, radiofrequency fields, and dirty electricity"

– Dr. Bruce Hoffman

It's worth considering how much we are affected by electromagnetic fields (EMFs), mobile signals, and Wi-Fi in our homes. This is a difficult one. I personally don't feel any differently when I put my phone in my pocket or when I don't. But would I sleep with a Wi-Fi router next to my head? Absolutely not.

EMFs are, unfortunately, all over the place. They come from the ever-increasing amount of tech we accumulate. That means every device that sends or receives signals, like Wi-Fi or a cell phone signal. But is this a particular problem when it comes to histamine intolerance? Let's look at the evidence:

1. Numerous studies link EMFs to increased mast cell activity and histamine release, although these cannot be described as conclusive. (17) In one fascinating study, the presence of histamine-containing mast

cells increased in volunteers sitting in front of TVs and computers. (18)

2. More papers, such as *A theoretical model based upon mast cells and histamine to explain humans' recently proclaimed sensitivity to electric and/or magnetic fields (19),* would be welcome.

3. More generally, some people experience an immediate difference in their energy levels when they cut their EMF exposure. Studies suggest that EMF exposure affects sleep and mood (20), although other scientists have argued that the evidence is weak.

Your brain may be beginning to fry at this point, and not because of EMFs. You might reasonably be wondering why the evidence appears so weak. It is admittedly unclear.

Studies like those referenced above suggest a potential link between mast cells and EMFs, but why is it inconclusive? One argument is that short-term EMF studies don't necessarily consider the cellular changes that could occur over much longer periods. So, I may not feel any different when I put my phone in my pocket today, but it might affect me over the long term?

My personal conclusion is that it is worth following steps to reduce your EMF exposure, both for histamine intolerance, and for general health.

Here are some suggestions. (These are the steps I follow)

- Use airplane mode as much as you can.
- Think carefully before putting your phone in your pocket or touching it to your ear.

- On that theme, use a mobile phone case that deflects the signal from your most sensitive areas. I use one made by Gadget Guard.
- Avoid putting your laptop on your lap, or get an EMF-blocking laptop pad. Defender Shield makes good ones.
- Use wired headphones. Don't use Bluetooth-connected earphones – this is especially important for children, whose developing brains are more vulnerable to electromagnetic radiation (21).
- Try hollow air tube headphones. These conduct the sound to your ears via sound waves using no metal. These tubes replace the traditional wires inside Bluetooth headphones and can reduce radiation by up to 99%. But the sound quality is inferior. I have a pair, but the music quality from these headphones is poor – I can't bring myself to listen to music that sounds that bad! So regulation Apple wired headphones it is.

You can dive even deeper – my friend Rich bought himself an EMF canopy. He draped this over his bed at night, akin to an exotic, high-tech mosquito net, blocking EMFs from a nearby train station. He's so fond of it that he even takes it on vacation. Miraculously, his wife has not divorced him.

Although the effects of EMF are widely debated, I've spoken to many experts during the research for this book and on my podcast, *Zestology*, who believe these steps are important. That's good enough for me, even if I don't take an EMF canopy on holiday with me.

Supplements and Medication

We are more than halfway through Part 2: *The Road To Recovery*, and you may be thinking – *why don't I just take antihistamines? After all, they are readily available over the counter, and with one pill, I can solve everything you've been discussing over the last three chapters?*

Good question. First of all, with medication and supplements, we're in the hands of your histamine-knowledgeable practitioner. With that acknowledged, they may well prescribe antihistamines, especially if your symptoms are very debilitating.. BUT... you may not want to be on these long-term.

In this section, we'll examine whether you should take; over-the-counter antihistamines, "natural" supplements such as Vitamin C, Zeolite, and methylated vitamins, or a mixture of both.

Remember, this book's content is for informational purposes only. Introducing supplements should be done with the help of a skilled practitioner. The following is purely based on my experience and research.

Antihistamines

Antihistamines have only been around since the 1930s, and at first, they were fairly ineffective. The scientific community scrambled to come up with new medicines that could help with allergies, and discoveries in the field came rapidly but haphazardly. (22)

For example, the first H1 receptor antagonist, thymo-ethyl-diethylamine, was invented in 1937. But it didn't work well and was way too toxic for humans. (Not a win-win, but a lose-lose – "Sorry, you still have your allergy symptoms, and now you've been poisoned too").

Regardless, as the Second World War approached, histamine pioneers were getting into their stride around the world. In particular, Dimenhydrinate (Dramamine) was starting to be tested as an antihistamine. And then scientists stumbled upon a peculiar discovery.

One patient who received the drug was a pregnant woman with a history of car sickness. But her symptoms miraculously vanished when she took dimenhydrinate a few minutes before getting on a tramcar. The placebo didn't work.

Then, researchers gave it to a considerable sample of American soldiers on a long and horrendously choppy boat trip to Germany in mid-winter. In an experiment known as "Operation Seasickness", the soldiers' participation was described as "involuntary..". Leaving aside the ethical violations involved in an involuntary experiment, the men who were given dimenhydrinate didn't get seasick. Conditions were so bad that the allergist in charge of the experiment described the soldiers who hadn't taken dimenhydrinate; "stretched out in semi-conscious condition on the floors until more seaworthy individuals managed to drag them to the sick bay or back to their hammocks. The latrines became temporarily indescribably repulsive." But not the ones who'd taken dimenhydrinate, although they did report getting rather drowsy. (23)

This unethical but successful experiment was hailed as a tremendous moment and the drug was available in stores that year. The antihistamine industry was born, turning out an enormous range of products that could treat everything from allergy symptoms, nausea, and motion sickness to schizophrenia. (24)

These days, of course, antihistamines are a massive business and are far more refined. They are (technical term alert) H1 histamine receptor antagonists. They intercept histamine molecules before they can bond with H1 receptors, effectively neutralizing symptoms caused by H1 receptor stimulation. That means they're often prescribed to ease the misery of hay fever, rashes, and allergies. These are the sort of symptoms those of us with histamine intolerance often suffer with.

They are less sleep-inducing these days. In fact, research continues to focus on creating even more effective and specific antihistamine drugs with fewer side effects. Antihistamines have become increasingly targeted, aiming to block specific histamine receptors, such as the H1 or H2 receptors, for more precise symptom control.

I bet you've come across some of the most famous antihistamines before. These hay fever meds are common. Some histamine-intolerance sufferers swear by over-the-counter medications (OTCs) like Loratadine as the only effective solution for flare-ups. (25)

I sometimes take these during May and June for seasonal allergies, but not the rest of the time. I find their use to be counter-productive long-term (and I don't want to be on any medication permanently). As always, this is just my experience. Some histamine-intolerant individuals have reported improvements from Loratadine and other OTCs, yet have found natural supplements more effective in the long run.

This is very much one for your doctor or practitioner. If you suffer from severe symptoms, you may need medication such as these OTCs and perhaps something more substantial. In the long term, you will probably want to be free of medication like me.

In addition, it should be acknowledged that antihistamines merely manage the symptoms of histamine intolerance, without addressing the underlying root cause.

A sticking plaster doesn't solve the problem.

Over time, the body may become more tolerant of these medications, reducing their effectiveness. Additionally, long-term use of antihistamines *may* lead to potential side effects, making them less suitable as a chronic solution for histamine intolerance. For instance, the potential side effects of Loratadine (26) are listed as:

- headache
- dry mouth
- nosebleed
- sore throat
- mouth sores
- difficulty falling asleep or staying asleep
- nervousness
- weakness
- stomach pain
- diarrhea
- red or itchy eyes
- rash
- hives
- itching
- swelling of the eyes, face, lips, tongue, throat, hands, arms, feet, ankles, or lower legs
- hoarseness
- difficulty breathing or swallowing
- wheezing

The irony, of course, is that these are precisely the kind of symptoms we want to avoid when managing our histamine intolerance. Another antihistamine – diphenhydramine – is also prescribed as a sleeping pill, which, to me, is a good reason to avoid it unless I actually want to use it as a sleeping pill. However, even then, I'd prefer to take some Vitamin C and CBD. Which moves us nicely along to taking supplements to help with our histamine issues.

Supplements

Supplements can help with histamine intolerance. I always prefer the natural approach to dealing with histamine intolerance and health issues, which is reflected below. Here is a list of supplements you can explore with the help of your practitioner; I'll explore each one in detail. For links to the brands I use, plus some discount codes, visit www.histamineintolerance.net/supplements

- Histamine Nutrients (for histamine support especially before meals)
- Toxpravent (for detox and potentially, flare-ups)
- Other binders (for detox and, potentially, flare-ups)
- Vitamin C (a 'natural' antihistamine)
- Probiota HistaminX (a histamine-friendly probiotic)
- Quercetin (can bring relief in a flare-up)
- SPMs (an anti-inflammatory secret agent)
- DAOfood Plus (before meals)
- NaturDAO (also before meals, suitable for vegans)
- HistaminX (for flare-ups)
- Pycnogenol (for allergy symptoms)
- Colostrum (for immunity)
- Grass Fed Kidney (for natural DAO before meals)
- Magnesium (for relaxation and flare-ups)

- Adrenal Support (to help reduce stress)
- CBD (for sleep and relaxation)
- Methylated vitamins (for detox and general health)

Histamine Nutrients (formerly Histamine Block Plus)

I have been using Histamine Nutrients for a long time, although note this supplement has changed name; it used to be called *Histamine Block Plus*. It's a helpful supplement to have in your pocket on a night out. The idea is you take it just before a high-histamine meal (or drink). Pop two about 15 minutes before you eat. It is a great help. I never go out without it now. (My friends roll their eyes when I take out my pill box at the dinner table, but hey, it works).

Histamine Nutrients is a comprehensive formula containing the histamine-metabolizing enzyme DAO. It includes additional histamine-processing nutrients to support total body histamine breakdown. It's not cheap, so I save it for when it is most needed.

Toxaprevent

Toxaprevent is owned by a company called Nouveau Health-care, and the owner, Dilkiran "Dilly" Kular, is hugely knowl-edgeable and passionate about histamines. He's had his own histamine issues (always a good motivator to learn more) and has been helpful on my podcast and with any questions people have about Toxaprevent.

I found one particular benefit to taking Toxaprevent. The tests they've carried out on histamine removal in the stomach are remarkable. It helped me detox. Many of my symptoms start in the gut, and this binder is well worth a go. I take it on an empty stomach with a flare-up and half an hour before a high-histamine meal. Research shows it removes most of the histamine from the gut. I recommend starting slowly, as always, under the care of your practitioner.

Other binders

If your symptoms are gut-related, I've found binders to be a game-changer, and not just Toxaprevent. They work by absorbing all the toxins in the gut and can quickly go to work on reducing symptoms. Initially, I found that activated coconut charcoal worked well. But it used to dehydrate me a little. Another fave of mine is BioToxin Binder by CellCore.

This (admittedly very expensive) binder suits me well and gets on with the job of soaking up the excess histamine in my gut. If you are like me and one of your histamine symptoms can be dehydration, you may want to reduce the dose. The recommended dose is three capsules a day. I take 20% of one capsule every other day, and that suits me fine.

Vitamin C

When you are dealing with intense histamine symptoms, taking 1000-1500mg of vitamin C can help a bit in calming you down. (I use the words 'a bit' advisedly; it's not a miracle cure, but then nothing is). Vitamin C is a natural antihistamine that is easy to find. A good liposomal Vitamin C is a must with histamine intolerance. I use this when I am having a flare-up. The interesting bit about this vitamin is that it is a cofactor for diamine oxidase. This is the final enzyme that helps in the breakdown of histamine.

I use Pure Health Liposomal Vitamin C for purity and bioavailability. It's mixed with Sea Buckthorn, which is a miracle ingredient, and I can pop the sachets in my backpack when I'm out and about, too.

Probiota HistaminX

Oh, the probiotics I used to take in the past, thinking I was doing myself good, when, actually, they were making my symptoms worse. However, ProBiota HistaminX is a probiotic supplement designed using histamine-friendly probiotics. So it is quite a find. It is from the same company as Histamine Nutrients, started by one of my favorite practitioners, Dr. Ben Lynch. They created it because many probiotics can cause more harm than good for histamine-heads. This one, though, contains entirely histamine-friendly strains of bacteria. I used to take this supplement daily. I stopped because it's expensive, and sometimes hard to source, plus I don't feel I need it anymore.

Quercetin

This can bring relief in a flare-up. This supplement suppresses the mast cells from releasing histamine. It is also a potent antioxidant. Fun Fact: Our histamine levels are often highest very early – around 4 am. I went through a phase of taking this in the middle of the night to ease these symptoms. Not very convenient, but it worked for a while. Yes, I am pretty extreme, and, happily, these days, I am not waking up to take supplements in the middle of the night.

SPMs (Specialized Pro-resolving Mediators)

If your histamine intolerance triggers inflammation, SPMs could be the secret weapon to help restore balance.

This is a relatively new area I've begun to delve into. SPMs are Specialized Pro-resolving Mediators and they're an excellent Omega 3 option. This is impressive considering our typical go-tos like fish oil or algae often contain high histamine levels.

But why do they work? Omega-3 fatty acids can be converted into Specialized Pro-resolving Mediators (SPMs) in the body. So you are cutting out the middleman by taking SPMs. They then play a crucial role in resolving inflammation, and as we know histamine intolerance often results in inflammation.

SPMs are a fascinating breakthrough, and come with a hefty price tag, but the potential benefits are worth the investment, at least for me.

Research is developing in relation to inflammation (27, 28); however, it is not histamine-specific. It is an area I'm particularly excited about, but it is one you must consult with your practitioner about.

DAOfood Plus

Another pre-meal DAO enzyme supplement. An effective tool to have in your biohacking arsenal and an alternative to other DAO supplements I've listed.

NaturDAO

So you want to take DAO enzyme, but you are vegan?

NaturDAO is a vegan supplemental source of DAO. It is made out of organic peas and lentils. I don't use this, but many people love it.

HistaminX

When histamine flare-ups strike, HistaminX can help. Contains stinging nettle extract, luteolin, rutin, quercetin, bromelain, and glucoraphanin. I used to take this regularly, but I now struggle to buy it in the UK for some reason. It is a unique blend that works to help your body manage these unexpected surges of histamine.

Pycnogenol

Made from tree bark. This plant extract can alleviate common allergy symptoms. Again, not a go-to for me, but many love it.

Grass Fed Kidney

Offering a natural source of DAO, Grass Fed Kidney is like the primal diet strategy, helping you handle histamine the way our ancestors might have. Might be particularly helpful if your histamine intolerance is genetic.

Magnesium

The jack-of-all-trades in the supplement world, magnesium helps with everything from relaxation to managing histamine flare-ups, optimizing body function, and helping with sleep. I use magnesium every day and find it helpful for histamine-related symptoms.

Adrenal Support

Stress can exacerbate histamine issues, which is where adrenal support supplements like Seeking Health Adrenal Nutrients come in. They can help reduce stress levels and get you back in balance.

CBD

Known for its calming effects, CBD can help at nighttime, promoting better sleep and relaxation. Some people react to particular brands of CBD, so, as with all these supplements, go slowly and test carefully, as well as making sure you get a reputable, well-tested brand that doesn't contain any THC.

Methylation and methylated vitamins

Many of us in the histamine intolerance community don't methylate very well. I'm in that camp, for sure. And when we start to methylate better, it could be the moment that our histamine symptoms begin to improve. But what the hell is methylation? Over to respected practitioner Chris Kresser.

"Methylation is a vital metabolic process that happens in every cell and every organ of our body. Life would simply not exist without it. It takes place more than a billion times per second in the body. That should give you some idea of how important methylation is. Anything that's happening a billion times per second is probably pretty crucial to our survival and well-being."

Thanks, Chris, for explaining it far better than I could.

Methylation issues often lead to histamine-related symptoms. They do in my case. But before you get too excited about methylated vitamins, a cautionary tale: When I first found out about methylation, I was so excited, I started taking max-dose methylation supplements. For two weeks, I felt incredible. Like, the best ever. There was a spring in my step, and I had so much energy. And then – I went through the worst crash. I was extremely nauseous and ill for two months. Two MONTHS.

My body was so excited at getting all these new nutrients that it started detoxing far too quickly. I then had a load of toxins swimming around in my system. (That's probably not the technical way of describing it, but there you go). So, be warned: Don't try this at home, folks.

Methylation should ideally be undertaken with the help of your doctor or practitioner, especially if you are histamine intolerant.

Methylation can often be quite an important piece of the puzzle. And methylation issues are sometimes related to genetics. I can tolerate normal-dose methylated supplements now, but it's taken me almost a decade to get there. Everyone's body is unique, and these supplements will work differently for everyone.

Always consult with your doctor or practitioner before starting any new supplement regimen, and, since I've mentioned this a lot, in the next section we'll be turning our attention to finding a practitioner who *really gets* histamine intolerance, and can help you to heal.

LOW-HISTAMINE LIFESTYLE AT-A-GLANCE

- ☐ **Consider your home and surroundings: check for mold, air quality, ad EMFs**
- ☐ **Review household items: identify common triggers like strong scents or chemicals**
- ☐ **Use apps and tech to help: *Think Dirty, EWG's Skin Deep* and *Yuka* are all helpful**
- ☐ **Consider symptom-managing supplements and antihistamines (in consultation with a professional**

7. Low-Histamine Advanced

"The part can never be well unless the whole is well."

– Plato

Have you ever tried to find an answer on Google, but it seemed like it just doesn't exist? That was my health journey for the longest time. I've sat in numerous clinics, filled out countless symptom forms, and shared my story with a parade of practitioners. All of them meant well, and many came highly recommended. They would listen, run tests, and suggest changes to my diet. Yet, they all missed something important: the role of histamine.

Navigating the world of health and wellness can be tough. Doctors, brilliant as they might be, often don't understand the nuances of histamine intolerance. And the few practitioners who do? They're like rare gems. The high demand for them means high prices. Unsurprisingly, it took me years and a decent chunk of change before someone finally connected the dots.

You might expect that, in our advanced world full of scientific knowledge, understanding something as important as histamine intolerance would be straightforward. However, I've learned that there's still much to discover. So, if you've felt better — lighter, clearer, and healthier — since reading this book and following the program, it's a sign you should explore this further.

Now, we're ready to take it to the next level. I want you to keep up with the positive changes you've already implemented in your diet, stress management, sleep routines, and overall lifestyle. These consistent efforts are key to building a strong foundation for long-term health and managing histamine intolerance effectively.

And then, in this chapter, a real focus is on finding the right practitioner. Yes, it might be expensive, but the value of someone who truly understands your situation cannot be overstated. Tackling this alone, no matter how much you know, is a big task. Many practitioners, I've noticed, lack extensive experience with histamine intolerance. That's why, before starting this important partnership, I'll provide you with a set of questions. These will help you to find a professional who really knows the details of histamine intolerance.

Why do I need to bother with a practitioner? Isn't the program you've suggested enough?

You've hopefully made huge strides over the course of this book already, but are you still wondering about the root cause of your histamine intolerance? WHY are you histamine intolerant? There has to be an underlying reason. Could it be related to your old diet, a gut imbalance, exposure to mold and mycotoxins, long Covid or perhaps it's hormonal or linked to menopause?

Even with the extensive knowledge you've amassed, solving this puzzle without an experienced practitioner can feel like trying to decode the plot twists in 'Stranger Things'. It's time to call in the professionals…

ESSENTIAL QUESTIONS FOR YOUR HISTAMINE INTOLERANCE SPECIALIST

What are their credentials?

Your practitioner must boast substantial qualifications and relevant experience. We've seen how complicated the area of genetic analysis can be. You need a proper expert. Look for certified Functional Medicine practitioners, naturopaths or doctors with the relevant knowledge.

Do they understand terms like SNPs, DAO, the Histamine Bucket and so on?

If they don't, they may be great practitioners, but they're not the ones for you right now. Move on.

How frequently do they update their knowledge?

The whole field of health and wellness, particularly histamine intolerance, is constantly evolving. Therefore, it's vital for your specialist to stay abreast of the latest research and practices. Why drive a beat-up old car with dodgy brakes from the 70s when you could drive the latest model?

Do they offer ongoing support?

Histamine intolerance is a condition that doesn't just pause between sessions. Your practitioner should be there to guide you even outside of formal appointments, ensuring continuity in your healing journey. This is the mark of an exceptional specialist – the ability to provide consistent feedback and support between appointments (within reason of course).

Are they accessible?

On that theme, accessibility is important. Sometimes you feel really, really crap with histamine intolerance. You don't want a practitioner who's going to take a month to answer your calls or queries.

Have they had tangible successes?

Request testimonials and details about previous clients. A lack of testimonials could be a red flag. You want to know, specifically, about other clients they've worked with on histamine intolerance, and to see/hear/read testimonials from them.

Is there rapport?

This may seem obvious , but do you get on with them? Do you like them? It's incredible how many people persevere with a health coach they don't particularly get on with or believe in. Once you've seen them once, ask yourself the question – did you feel like it was worthwhile and you connected with them? If not, perhaps it's time to change and work with someone else. Sometimes the Tinder "swipe left" approach is needed until you find someone you click with.

What is their reputation and experience like?

Does your specialist have a solid standing in their field? How many years' of experience do they have? Your health is at stake, so it is worth working with somebody with experience and knowledge.

How do they utilize technology?

Modern healthcare is teaming up with technology. This isn't a must-have, but is your specialist leveraging this surge in health tech? And how? Healthcare is changing quickly. (This might be something like the latest in genetic analysis, updated mycotoxin tests, wearable health tech or CGMs – continuous glucose monitors – and lots else besides.

To round off this section, I can certainly recommend finding an excellent practitioner. I have one myself, and it makes a massive difference to me. I couldn't have healed in the way I have without one.

Advanced FAQs

Now it's time for some advanced histamine intolerance FAQs as we get towards the end of our program. As always, this is intended for educational and informational value, and you should speak to your practitioner before making any changes.

What about coffee? Can I still drink it?

The issue of coffee and histamine intolerance is the one I've been asked about more than any other over the past few years. Nobody wants to give up caffeine (at least not me).

Generally speaking, the idea is to try not to worry too much about each individual food and drink – honestly, life works better when we're not obsessing. But as we know, with histamine intolerance, sometimes we just *react*. Coffee is one of those things that divide opinion.

Coffee gets a big fat *thinking emoji* over on our site. Many love it and are fine with it. Others can tolerate the occasional cup, and I'm sorry to tell you that many more can't tolerate it without their histamine symptoms flaring up. It can be quite dehydrating, exacerbating the feelings of thirst and dehydration that people with histamine intolerance already get. And there is a big issue with mycotoxins in coffee too. Mycotoxins are toxic compounds produced by molds in food and drink, which can worsen our histamine intolerance, as we've seen. Over to coffee specialist Alex Higham:

"Molds and mycotoxins can be a big issue for all of us, if ignored. And there's a lot of evidence to point towards coffee being a significant contributor to our overall exposure to them."

I completely gave up coffee for 18 months, and I did feel better. But I missed it so much. When I reintroduced it, I found I could tolerate it again, and, let me tell you, that first coffee back was like pure rocket fuel.

However, I'm pretty sure if you are reading this Coffee FAQ, you will not want to give it up for 18 months, so here are some things you can do, with reference to what I do myself.

1. Mold-free and mycotoxin-free coffee seem to help. These are priced at a premium as they are rigorously tested. People often report they don't get the same sort of jitters from them they do from regular coffee. Try coffee companies like Alex Higham's Exhale Coffee (UK) or Purity Coffee and Danger Coffee (US).
2. Go organic if possible. As you might have guessed, mold-free, mycotoxin-free, organic coffee costs more than average, but you get what you pay for.

3. Avoid instant powdered coffee. The way instant powdered coffee is created is a chemical process that may not agree with your histamine intolerance. However, some organic freeze-dried instant brands may suit you better.

4. Avoid plastic capsules from machines (for example Nespresso). I completely avoided these for a long time as I felt they aggravated my symptoms. Now, I will have the occasional coffee from a machine, if that's all that is on offer, and (as with many other things. I'm not sure whether it affects me anymore.

5. Again, this is something you'll read more than once in this book, but if you suspect coffee is aggravating your symptoms, try taking DAO tablets beforehand and see if that helps. Good options might be Histamine Nutrients or NaturDAO. There are some other options elsewhere in this book.

6. Be realistic. Ultimately, as much as you have an intimate relationship with caffeine, if it's making your symptoms flare up, it's not worth it. Be realistic and cut it out if needed. This is not divorce. It's just a little time apart!

Should I drink tap water?

Living in this day and age, we're fortunate to have access to treated water that is free of harmful bacteria, parasites, and other nasties. However, the chemicals used to purify tap water might not fit well with our physiology, particularly for those of us dealing with histamine intolerance. The water we generally presume clean can be affected by the treatment employed to remove contaminants and other harmful byproducts. (29, 30)

In addition, tap water often contains contaminants that can have a long-term effect on our health. For example, the Environmental

Working Group in America found 171 times the recommended amount of arsenic in the tap water in Los Angeles.

When managing histamine intolerance, dehydration can be a particular symptom, so you might think hard about water. I believe it is also important to focus on the quality of water you're using to hydrate. This is where a solid water filter comes into play.

The market is flooded with water filters of all shapes and sizes. Filter jugs, bottles, taps, whole house filtration systems – you name it, they're available at your local supermarket, hardware store, or just a click away online. But (how can I put this politely) not all of them match up to my expectations.

Here's an interesting fact: Berkey Filters are popular with preppers, who prepare for extreme situations like natural disasters. These filters can purify even untreated water, removing almost all harmful bacteria and viruses. But don't worry, I'm not expecting an apocalypse anytime soon!

Also, third-party tests have shown impressive results, especially regarding arsenic in tap water (an increasing issue due to pollution). Berkey filters can eliminate over 99.9% of arsenic.

As water technology evolves, we see a range of options emerging. For instance, the LARQ bottle uses UV light to clean and sterilize water, offering a more affordable approach. On the more expensive end of the spectrum is AquaTru, which is popular with many.

Switching from tap water to filtered water won't instantly cure histamine intolerance, but it's a step in the right direction. I always notice the chlorine taste in tap water, which I don't enjoy. With a Berkey, (or another filter), that's not an issue. You'll get cleaner water, free from the chlorine taste. It's a long-term investment in managing your histamine intolerance and overall health.

Should I get Botox if I have histamine intolerance?

This may seem a surprising question, but it is one that has come up many times over on the site and social media.

Botox works by blocking the release of acetylcholine, a neurotransmitter responsible for muscle contractions. This leads to temporary muscle paralysis and, subsequently (for cosmetic reasons), a reduction in the appearance of wrinkles.

Let's start with the science, which seems hopeful (although don't get your hopes too high). A study published in the Journal of Dermatological Science in 2019 found that botulinum toxin could actually suppress the release of inflammatory mediators, including histamine, from human mast cells (31).

So, you might wonder if Botox could help with histamine intolerance symptoms. Unfortunately, from my experience, it's not that straightforward. I've heard from many people who've encountered significant issues with Botox, leading to extended histamine flare-ups that sound unpleasant. Obviously, this is anecdotal, although it is based on my experience of running the largest histamine intolerance website and social media. I'm open to being corrected about Botox, but for now, I'm choosing to age naturally. Please speak to your doctor on this one.

What about tattoos and histamine?

Let's talk about tattoos and their potential impact on histamine levels. I have one slightly crap tattoo from a long time ago. One day, I'll post a picture of it, but today is not the day. It makes me wonder, did that tattoo unknowingly trigger my histamine symptoms?

Tattooing involves injecting ink into the dermis layer of the skin, creating a permanent design. The body's immune system usually does react to it in some way – a normal reaction might be swelling and the skin feeling slightly itchy. But for those particularly sensitive to histamine, how significant is the immune response, including inflammation and histamine release?

Some of my followers report problems after getting a tattoo, ranging from a week-long itch to months of raised, itchy skin, especially if their histamine bucket is already high. Others experience no issues at all. Histamine intolerance really is unpredictable. I've struggled to back this up with science relating specifically to histamine, so we unfortunately have to file it under "anecdotal" at the moment. There are more general studies around tattoo sensitivity that may be of interest. (32,33) This is another one to run by your (histamine-intolerance-sympathetic) doctor or practitioner.

Two interesting suggestions from followers: One recommended testing the tattoo ink with a small dot on a hidden area to check for reactions. Smart idea. Another takes DAO enzyme pills before getting a tattoo as a precaution.

Is it possible that exercise might make my histamine intolerance symptoms worse rather than better?

It seems that exercise can sometimes trigger an acute histamine response, but how this works needs further exploration.

Studies including *Exercise-induced allergies: the Role of Histamine Release* (34) and *The Intriguing Role of Histamine in Exercise Responses* (35) have investigated this, but there is a need for more up-to-date, extensive studies and more in-depth work. The connection between histamine and exercise is without doubt real, but exactly what is going on is still unclear.

"Despite recent advances in determining the role of histamine in exercise responses, relatively little is known about this molecule in the context of exercise physiology, but it appears to be a fundamental component of exercise responses in humans." (35)

Many people have contacted me to say that sometimes they feel worse after heavy exercise, particularly during a flare-up. It is not a significant symptom for me, but I have previously perceived a subtle intensification post-exercise. (As always with histamine intolerance, I wasn't sure if this was symptom-related or just me being tired). If you notice a similar pattern, it is worth discussing personally with your practitioner, as there seems to be enough evidence to merit further investigation.

Do ice baths help when you are histamine intolerant?

Ice baths have become increasingly popular, due to their perceived health and resilience benefits. However, be mindful that the stress response triggered by cold exposure sometimes seems to be a bit overwhelming for those with histamine issues.

Currently, there isn't extensive research directly connecting ice baths or cold exposure to histamine intolerance. Nonetheless, many who've contacted me say that such intense cold can stress their body too much, and not everyone responds well to it.

In the past, I engaged in ice baths when my histamine levels were manageable, and I felt stable. Nowadays, since I moved to Portugal's milder climate, I prefer sea swimming, which has been a fantastic alternative. The sea here is cold, which means it's sometimes a sea dunk, rather than a sea swim. However it is not as extreme as an ice bath, making it a much better fit for managing my histamine intolerance.

LOW-HISTAMINE ADVANCED AT-A-GLANCE

☐ **Find the Right Practitioner: Choose someone who understands histamine intolerance well**

☐ **Consider Lifestyle Factors: Pay attention to coffee consumption, exercise, and cold exposure**

☐ **Review Overlooked Factors: Botox and water quality can influence symptoms**

☐ **Maintain Consistency: Keep up positive diet, stress management, and lifestyle changes**

PART 3

LOW-HISTAMINE SURVIVAL KIT: ESSENTIAL RESOURCES AND TOOLS

8. Ingredient List

This list is adapted from The Histamine Intolerance Site. It uses a tick/cross system to create a comprehensive, alphabetical histamine intolerance list. (On the website we use emojis but they don't work so well in a book.) Here's how it works:

- A tick (✓) indicates foods that our sources generally agree tend to be low-histamine
- A tick/cross combo (✓/✗) indicates foods that are medium histamine, or where there is debate about histamine levels
- A cross (✗) indicates foods that our sources seem to think are high-histamine

DISCLAIMER: Always check with your doctor or health practitioner before starting any new diet. This list is not advice; it is intended for information and discussion only.

Please note that you may disagree with some of the following. Histamine intolerance is specific for each person, and many sites differ wildly in their recommendations. There are so many controversial food items in histamine intolerance. Beef, chocolate, cacao, eggs, and berries seem to trigger conflicting opinions on the major sites. Again, this list is intended to be used in conjunction with your practitioner.

I am aware there are certain contradictions in this list. That's because every histamine food list contains confusing contradictions, and as best I can, I've tried to simplify. You'll probably find something you disagree with in this list – everybody disagrees, and that's why histamine intolerance truly is the WTF of health issues. So, I've worked hard to do the best I can.

I've consulted what I believe to be the best, most trusted resources on histamine intolerance (listed below – they still conflict, though!) and compiled what is currently (but by no means definitively) the best low-histamine diet list. This page aims to collate our most trusted sites and best knowledge, but please do your own testing. Let me know if you think anything is incorrectly listed below, and we can investigate further. When I refer to foods that are high in histamine, for ease, this also refers to foods that are histamine-releasing –even though there is a distinction.

Remember, this list is not forever. As you start to manage your histamine intolerance, there's a good chance you'll be able to welcome back some of your favorite foods. Stay hopeful, patient, and open to change.

Sources:

The Histamine Intolerance Site (our site has become a go-to list for checking histamine levels in food and drink when on the go)

Swiss Interest Group Histamine Intolerance (SIGHI) (pdf – the most comprehensive list, which breaks down histamine liberators, histamine blockers and high-histamine foods, and yet still has quite a few contradictions)

https://www.histamine-sensitivity.com/histamine_joneja.html (the excellent Janice Joneja on histamine)

Dr Axe on Histamine (a very helpful overview of Histamine Intolerance)

http://mthfr.net/histamine-intolerance-mthfr-and-methyla-tion/2015/06/11/ (Dr. Ben Lynch – brilliant on histamine and genes)

https://www.amymyersmd.com/2017/10/histamine-intoler-ance/ (Amy Myers – also very

useful on histamine)

https://www.bbcgoodfood.com/howto/guide/top-20-low-his-tamine-foods (low-histamine foods by registered nutritionist Kerry Torrens)

The List

acerola ✓

agave syrup ✓

alcohol ✗

alcoholic beverages ✗

algae and algae derivatives ✗

almond ✓/✗ (a few almonds seem to be okay for many, a tub of almond butter not so!)

amaranth ✓

anchovies ✗

anise, aniseed ✓/✗

apple ✓

apple cider vinegar ✓/✗

apricot ✓

artichoke ✓

artificial sweeteners ✗

Asimina triloba ✓/✗

asparagus ✓

aubergine ✗

avocado ✗

bamboo shoots ✓/✗

banana ✗

Barbary fig ✓/✗

barley ✓/✗

barley malt, malt ✗

basil ✓

bay laurel, laurel ✓/✗

beans (pulses) ✗

beef (depending on the age of the beef, organic, freshly cooked) ✓/✗

beef (fresh) ✓

beer ✗

beetroot ✓

bell pepper (hot) ✗

bell pepper (sweet) ✓

bison (organic, freshly cooked) ✓

bivalves (mussels, oyster, clams, scallops) ✗

black caraway ✓

black caraway oil ✓

blackberry ✓

blackcurrants ✓

blue cheeses, mold cheeses (nb, one of the absolute worst!) ✗

blue fenugreek ✗

blueberries ✓

bok choy ✓

borlotti beans ✗

bouillon (because of yeast extract/meat extract/gluta-mate) ✗

boysenberry ✓/✗

brandy ✗

Brazil nut ✓

bread ✓/✗

broad bean ✗

broad-leaved garlic ✓/✗

broccoli ✓

brown algae, algae ✗

brussels sprouts ✓/✗

buckrams ✓/✗

buckwheat ✗

butter (usually okay) ✓

butterkäse ✓

buttermilk (slightly sour, starting to ferment) ✗

cabbage, green or white (except cauliflower and kohlrabi) ✓

cactus pear ✓/✗

caraway ✓

cardamom ✓

carrot ✓

cashew nut ✓/✗ (go very cautiously – some tolerate cashews, I'm not one of those people)

cassava ✓

cassava flour ✓

cauliflower ✓

celery ✓

celery cabbage ✓

cep ✗

chamomile tea ✓

champagne ✗

chard stalks ✓/✗

chayote ✓/✗

cheddar cheese ✗

cheese made from unpasteurised "raw" milk ✗

cheese: soft cheeses ✓/✗ (these are tolerated much better than hard cheese, introduce them cautiously)

cheese: hard cheese, all well matured cheeses ✗

cherry ✓

chestnut, sweet chestnut ✓

chia ✓

chicken (organic, freshly cooked) ✓

chicken (must be fresh, not leftovers) ✓

chickpeas ✗

chicory ✓

chili pepper, red, fresh ✗

chives ✓/✗

chocolate ✗ (sad times – white chocolate may be slightly better tolerated)

cilantro ✓/✗

cinnamon ✓/✗

citrus fruits ✗

clover ✗

cloves ✓

Coca-Cola ✓/✗

cocoa butter ✓/✗

cocoa drinks ✗

cocoa, cocoa powder (chocolate, etc.) ✗

coconut fat, coconut oil ✓

coconut, coconut shavings, coconut milk ✓

coffee ✓/✗ (see Chapter 7: *Low-Histamine Advanced* for lots more on coffee)

Coke ✓/✗

cola-drinks ✓/✗

common sea-buckthorn ✓

coriander ✓

corn ✓

corn salad, lamb's lettuce ✓

cornflakes (if there are no additives) ✓

courgette ✓

cowberry ✓

crab ✗

cranberry ✓

cranberry nectar ✓

crawfish ✗

crayfish ✗

cream cheeses (this means very young cheeses), plain, without additives ✓/✗

cream, sweet, without additives ✓

cress: garden cress ✓/✗

cucumber ✓

cumin ✗

curd cheese ✓/✗

curry ✓/✗

dates (dried, desiccated) ✓/✗

dextrose ✓

dill ✓/✗

distilled white vinegar ✓

dog rose ✓/✗

dragon fruit, pitaya ✓

dried meat (any kind) ✗

dry-cured ham ✗

duck ✓

duck (organic, freshly cooked) ✓

earth almond ✓

egg white ✓/✗

egg yolk ✓/✗

eggplant ✗

eggs, chicken egg, whole egg ✗

elderflower cordial ✓

endive ✓

energy drinks ✗

entrails ✗

espresso ✓/✗ (see Chapter 7: *Low-Histamine Advanced* on coffee)

ethanol ✗

ewe's milk, sheep's milk ✓

extract of malt ✗

farmer's cheese (a type of fresh cheese) ✓

fennel ✓

fennel flower (Nigella sativa) ✓

fennel flower oil (Nigella sativa) ✓

fenugreek ✗

feta cheese ✓/✗

figs (fresh or dried) ✓/✗

fish (Freshly caught within an hour or frozen within an hour is considered to be the only low-histamine fish. See Chapter 4: *Low-Histamine Diet* for more.) ✓

fish (in the shop in the cooling rack, on ice, or any other fish) ✗

Flaxseed (linseed) ✓

Fontina cheese ✗

fructose (fruit sugar) ✓

game ✓/✗

garden cress ✓/✗

garlic ✓/✗ (this is usually well tolerated)

Geheimratskaese, Geheimrats cheese ✓

German turnip ✓/✗

ginger ✓
glucose ✓
goat's milk, goat milk ✓
goji berry, Chinese wolfberry, Chinese boxthorn, Himalayan goji, Tibetan goji ✓
goose (organic, freshly cooked) ✓
gooseberry, gooseberries ✓
Gouda cheese (young) ✓/✗
Gouda cheese, old ✗
gourds ✓
grapefruit ✗
grapes ✓
green algae, algae ✗
green beans ✓/✗
green peas ✓/✗
green split peas ✓/✗
green tea ✓/✗
guava ✗
ham (dried, cured) ✗
hazelnut ✓/✗
hemp seeds (Cannabis sativa) ✓
herbal teas with medicinal herbs (this depends how many ingredients and the tea blend – a source of great debate) ✓/✗
honey ✓

horseradish ✓/✗
hot chocolate ✗
Indian fig opuntia, Barbary fig, cactus pear, spineless cactus, prickly pear, tuna ✓/✗
innards ✗
inverted sugar syrup ✓
ispaghula, psyllium seed husks ✓
Jeera ✗
jostaberry ✓
juniper berries ✓
kaki ✓
kale ✓
kefir ✗
kelp (large seaweeds (algae) belonging to the brown algae) ✗
kelp, seaweed, algae ✗
Khorasan wheat ✓
kiwi fruit ✗
kohlrabi ✓/✗
Kombu seaweed ✗
lactose (milk sugar) ✓
lady finger banana ✓/✗
lamb (organic, freshly cooked) ✓
lamb's lettuce, corn salad ✓
langouste ✗
lard ✓

laurel, bay laurel, sweet bay, bay tree, true laurel ✓/✗

leek ✓/✗

lemon ✗

lemon peel, lemon zest ✗

lemonade ✓/✗

lentils ✗

lettuce, iceberg ✓

lettuce: head and leaf lettuces ✓

lime ✗

lime blossom tea, limeflower, flowers of large-leaved lime tree ✓

lingonberry ✓

liquor, clear ✗

liquor, schnapps, spirits, cloudy (not colorless) ✗

liquorice root ✗

lobster ✗

loganberry ✓/✗

lychee ✓

macadamia ✓/✗

malt extract ✗

malt, barley malt ✗

maltodextrin ✓ (test extremely cautiously. Other lists seem to think maltodextrin doesn't affect histamine levels; personally I'm not so sure.)

maltose, malt sugar (pure) ✓

mandarin orange ✗

mango ✓/✗

maple syrup ✓

margarine (regardless of histamine levels, this stuff is not optimal for health) ✗

marrow ✓

Mascarpone cheese ✓/✗

mate tea ✓/✗

meat extract ✗

melons (except watermelon) ✓

meridian fennel ✓

milk, lactose free ✓/✗

milk, pasteurized ✓

milk, UHT ✓

milk powder ✓/✗

millet ✓

minced meat (if eaten immediately after its production) ✓

minced meat (open sale or pre-packed) ✗

mineral water, still ✓

mint ✓

mold cheeses✗

monosodium ascorbate ✓

morel ✗

morello cherries ✓

Mozzarella cheese ✓/✗

mulberry ✓/✗

mung beans (germinated, sprouting) ✓/X

mushrooms, different types ✓/X

mustard, mustard seeds, mustardseed powder X

napa cabbage ✓

nashi pear ✓/X

nectarine ✓/X

Nigella sativa oil ✓

Nigella sativa seed ✓

non-organic meat – this is all suspect, especially if aged X

Nori seaweed X

nut grass ✓

nutmeg ✓/X

nutmeg flower ✓

nutmeg flower oil ✓

nuts ✓/X

oat drink, oat milk ✓/X

oats ✓

olive oil ✓

olives ✓/X

onion ✓/X (this is usually well tolerated)

orange X

orange juice X

orange peel, orange zest X

oregano ✓

ostrich ✓

ostrich (organic, freshly cooked) ✓

oyster X

pak choi ✓

palm kernel oil ✓

palm oil, dendê oil ✓

palm sugar ✓

papaya, pawpaw X

paprika, hot X

paprika, sweet ✓

parsley ✓

parsnip ✓

passionfruit

pasta (search individual ingredients, eg wheat ✓/X, corn ✓)

paw paw ✓/X

peach ✓

peanuts X

pear ✓/X

pear, peeled canned in sugar syrup ✓/X

pearl sago ✓

peas (green) ✓/X

pea shoots ✓

pepper, black X

pepper, white X

peppermint tea ✓

perennial wall-rocket X

Persian cumin ✓

persimmon ✓

pickled cabbage ✗

pickled cucumber ✗

pickled gherkin ✗

pickled vegetables ✗

pine nuts ✓/✗

pineapple ✗

pistachio ✓/✗

pitaya, pitahaya, dragon fruit ✓

plum ✓/✗

pomegranate ✓

poppy seeds ✓/✗

porcini mushroom ✗

pork (organic, freshly cooked) ✓

potato with peel ✓

potato, new, with peel ✓

potato, peeled ✓

poultry meat ✓

prawn ✗

prickly pear ✓/✗

processed cheese ✗

products made from unprocessed (raw) milk ✗

prune ✓/✗

Prunus domestica subsp. Domestica ✓/✗

psyllium seed husks ✓

pulses (soy, beans, lentils... some other pulses are listed individually, always test) ✗

pumpkin seed oil ✓

pumpkin seeds ✓

pumpkins (various varieties) ✓

purple granadilla, passionfruit ✓/✗

quail ✓

quail (organic, freshly cooked) ✓

quail eggs ✓

quark ✓

quince ✓

quinine ✓/✗

quinoa ✓

rabbit (organic, freshly cooked) ✓

raclette cheese ✗

radish: red radish (the tiny red round ones) ✓

radish: white radish (the long white ones) ✓

raisins (if no sulfur) ✓

ramsons ✓/✗

rapeseed oil (called canola oil in US) ✓

raspberry ✗

raw milk ✓

ready made cheese preparations ✗

red algae, algae ✗

red cabbage ✓

red wine vinegar ✗

redcurrants, currant ✓

rhubarb ✓/✗

rice ✓

rice biscuits, rice cakes ✓

rice krispies ✓

rice milk, rice drink ✓/✗

rice noodles ✓

Ricotta cheese ✓/✗

Rochefort cheese ✗

rock lobsters ✗

Roman coriander ✓

Roman coriander oil ✓

rooibos tea ✓

Roquefort cheese ✓/✗

rose hip ✓/✗

rosemary ✓

rum ✗

rye ✓/✗

safflower oil ✓

sage ✓

sage tea ✓

sago ✓

salami ✗

sallow thorn ✓

salmon ✗ (see Fish section in Chapter 4: *Low-Histamine Diet*. Only considered low-histamine if freshly caught and eaten within an hour or frozen at sea)

sauerkraut ✗

sausages of all kinds ✗

Savoy cabbage ✓/✗

schnapps, clear (colorless) ✗

seafood, sea food ✗

seasoning made of hydrolysated proteins ✗

seaweed, seaweed ✗

seaweeds and seaweed derivatives ✗

sesame ✓/✗

sharon fruit ✓

sheep's milk, sheep milk ✓

shellfish ✗

shrimp ✗

smoked fish (any) ✗

smoked meat (any) ✗

snow peas ✓/✗

soda ✓/✗

soft cheese ✓/✗ (tend to be tolerated much better than hard cheese, introduce cautiously) soft drinks ✓/✗

sour cherry ✓

sourcream ✓/✗

soy (soy beans, soy flour) ✗

soy milk, soy drink ✗

soy sauce ✗

sparkling wine ✗

spelt ✓

spinach ✗

spineless cactus ✓/✗

spiny lobsters ✗

spirit vinegar ✓

spirits, clear (colorless) ✗

squashes ✓

star anise, star anise seed, Chinese star anise, badiam ✓/✗

starch ✓

stevia ✓

stinging nettle ✗

stinging nettle herbal tea ✓/✗

strawberry ✗

sucrose ✓

sugar (beet sugar, cane sugar) ✓

sugar banana ✓/✗

sunflower oil ✓/✗

sunflower seeds ✗

sweetcorn ✓

sweet potato ✓

tamarillo, Solanum betaceum ✓/✗

tap water ✓ (we much prefer filtered – use the Berkey water filter)

tea, black tea ✗

thyme, common thyme, German thyme, garden thyme ✓

tiger nut sedge ✓

tomato ✗

tomato juice ✗

tongue (veal, beef) ✓

trifolium ✗

trigonella ✗

trout ✓/✗

tuna ✗

turkey ✓

turkey (organic, freshly cooked) ✓

turmeric ✓

turnip ✓/✗

turnip cabbage ✓/✗

vanilla extract ✓/✗ (beware vanilla in alcohol tincture)

vanilla, vanilla pod, vanilla powder, vanilla sugar ✓/✗

veal (fresh) ✓

venison ✓/✗

verbena herbal tea ✓

vinegar: apple cider vinegar ✓/✗ (better tolerated than other vinegars)

vinegar: balsamic vinegar ✗

vinegar ✗

Wakame seaweed ✗

walnut ✗

walnut oil ✗

watercress ✓

watermelon ✓/✗

wheat ✓/✗

wheat germ ✗

whey ✓

white button mushroom ✓/✗

white onion ✓/✗

white vinegar, spirit vinegar ✓

white wine vinegar ✗

wild garlic ✓/✗

wild meat ✓/✗

wild rice ✓

wine ✗ (check out the Low Histamine Wine Club online. I'm still skeptical but it might work for you)

wine: red wine ✗

wine: Schilcherwein ✗

wine: white wine ✗

wood garlic ✓/✗

yam ✓

yeast (fresh, dried, in all forms) ✓/✗

yeast extract ✗

yellow nutsedge ✓

yellow split peas ✓/✗

yogurt/yoghurt ✗

zucchini (courgettes) ✓

9. Food Polls: Entirely Unscientific (But Quite Useful)

Building upon the comprehensive food list, let's venture into something a bit different: my Entirely Unscientific (But Quite Useful) Food Polls.

Navigating the complex world of histamine intolerance can be challenging, especially with so many ✓/✗ foods. As we know, the uncertainty stems from lots of factors: fluctuating histamine levels in foods, varying individual reactions, limited research and testing, and wildly differing opinions on histamine levels in food. This ambiguity raises the question: how can we make sense of it all?

Enter the Food Polls. Over the years, I've engaged my social media followers in polls to gather insights on those seemingly random and contradictory medium-rated foods. While they are not scientifically rigorous, they offer valuable, real-world perspectives. Remember, just because they're not conducted in a lab doesn't strip them of their usefulness.

These polls are a collective effort, in which I ask numerous people to share their experiences with specific foods. They should be viewed as an informal guide, a conversation starter with your practitioner, and a source of communal learning. I always approach the results with a pinch of salt, combining them with my own testing.

The format has varied from simple yes/no votes to more nuanced options, which have evolved as Instagram developed more sophisticated polling.

Personally, the insights from these polls have been useful. For example, nutritional yeast emerged as a potential histamine trigger for me, something I had never considered before. These revelations can lead to further investigation and personal experimentation.

There are surprises too. Take sushi, for example. I still steer clear of it, despite a nearly even split in the poll results, showing that many with histamine intolerance still enjoy it. The only sushi I eat these days are the boring ones with the cucumber in the middle, with no soy sauce!

Remember, use these polls as a bit of fun, an informal guide in your histamine journey.

The Food Polls

Food Item	%✓	%X	%✓/X
apples	80	20	
Athletic Greens (AG1) powder	38	62	
banana	33	67	
BBQ Seasoning	19	59	22
BCAA supplements	32	17	51
beef chili, no beans	50	50	

buckwheat	49	51	
cashew	37	63	
cassava flour	76	24	
CBD gummies	60	40	
cheddar cheese	35	65	
chickpeas	36	64	
cinnamon	51	49	
coconut	74	26	
coconut aminos	64	36	
coconut oil	66	18	16
coffee	56	44	
cottage cheese/quark	60	40	
crisps cooked with sunflower oil	40	43	17
curry powder	42	58	
double cream	42	58	
dragon fruit	67	33	
eggs	58	22	20
feta	56	44	

gooseberries	59	41	
kale	72	28	
latte (coffee with milk)	43	35	22
macadamia nuts	70	30	
mango	76	24	
matcha tea	36	34	30
mozzarella	76	24	
mushrooms	46	54	
nutmeg	56	44	
nutritional yeast	34	66	
oats	74	26	
olive oil	93	7	
oranges	22	56	22
organic meat	91	9	
papaya	36	64	
peach	80	20	
pears	72	28	
peas	58	42	
pine nuts	61	39	
popcorn	51	20	29

potatoes	85	15	
psyllium husk	71	29	
pumpkin seeds	76	24	
quinoa	73	27	
raspberries	62	38	
red peppers	62	23	15
roast potatoes	83	10	7
rocket	77	23	
salmon from frozen	60	40	
seaweed, edible	52	48	
sushi	45	55	
white chocolate	55	45	

10. Histamine-Friendly Products and Services

This is a list of the many products, services, books and practices I have used in connection with histamine intolerance. Some have direct relevance to reducing histamine levels, and some are more generally related to health. I've explained why I've included them in this book in each entry.

In the eBook version of this book, the list has hyperlinks. If you are reading this in paperback, head to www.histamineintolerance.net, where you can download this free directory via a pdf with hyperlinks.

In some instances, this directory includes discounts (which are often quite large). As always, consult your practitioner before starting anything new.

- 23andme – genetic testing. Helpful for histamine intolerance.
- 40 Years Of Zen – for the deepest possible dive into neurofeedback. This was useful for me to reduce stress, which impacts histamine levels. However, it is pricey.
- Air Angel – an air purifier from HypoAir that kills 99 percent of allergens, odors, germs, and viruses, including various forms of coronavirus. It was successfully tested on SARS-CoV-2 (the Covid-19 virus). It's excellent if you get a stuffed-up nose, and lots of us with histamine intolerance do. Other recommended purifiers include Air Doctor. See the special section on air purifiers earlier in the book.

- Berkey Water Filter – removes 99.9999999% of pathogenic bacteria and 99.999% of viruses while leaving the essential minerals your body needs – thi is a great healthy water hack. Good hydration is necessary with histamine intolerance, as sufferers report getting thirsty and dehydrated more often. Certainly, that's the case with me.
- Binaural beats app – reduce stress = reduce your histamine levels. This is proven to induce altered states of consciousness, such as an Alpha state (reducing stress and anxiety – a proper chill-out zone) or a Gamma state (the ideas zone – for memory processing, language, and learning).
- Blue-blocking glasses – important for sleep (and we've examined the links between sleep and histamine). There are lots of options, but these are one of the brands I use.
- Blue-blocking USB light from Bon Charge – we have these all around the house. It has a brilliant design and a lovely red glow to help you sleep at night. I consider this critical with histamine intolerance.
- Bulletproof Charcoal – activated charcoal binds to toxins and helps get rid of them. Pure Health is a UK-based brand that provides a good product. (Their Liposomal Vitamin C is also great for a histamine flare-up).
- Dan Harris's 10% Happier app – a good meditation app. It is good for reducing stress, which is important with histamine levels.
- DAOfood Plus – a supplement that provides DAO, the primary enzyme that degrades ingested histamine. Also contains Vitamin C and Quercetin.
- Daylio – an effective symptom and lifestyle tracking app. This works well because it's so simple. It takes

seconds to fill out every evening and is a fully customizable tracking app based on mood. They say, "Create some useful habits like running, eating more healthily or waking up earlier." Not perfect, but very helpful.

- Exhale Coffee – good organic, low-mycotoxin, low-mold coffee, with a nice taste. A great low-histamine option.
- Evergreen – remember how I said plastic coffee capsules triggered my histamine issues? These are stainless steel capsules to put your coffee in, compatible with Nespresso®, Dolce Gusto® and others. A nice idea.
- EWG's Skin Deep site – search for all your personal care products and find out if they are clean and safe. This is crucial for histamine intolerant people, as products high in fragrance, artificial scent, or artificial/ toxic ingredients can quickly trigger us.
- Exist – a behavior change app with which you can track everything together. Understand your behavior.
- F:Lux – a free download that warms up your computer display at night to match your indoor lighting. Sleep hygiene is important with histamine intolerance. Apple products (and other computers) have in-built products that perform a similar function.
- Found My Fitness – analyzes DNA testing and has a specific histamine section and many other great health resources. Learn more about your genes and histamine intolerance.
- Freestyle Libre – a Continuous Glucose Monitor (CGM) that lasts 14 days. It might be helpful for histamine intolerance. I found it useful to identify the effect of seed oils on my glucose levels, but that may or may not be directly linked to histamine issues.
- Gadget Guard – a phone case snappily described as "the world's only case with patented technology

proven to reduce cell phone radiation by up to 75% while maintaining signal strength". See the section on EMFs and histamine issues.

- Get A Drip – pumps in high strength Vitamin C and hydration. It always alleviates my histamine symptoms. This particular company is London-based, but you can find them worldwide. Unfortunately, it is not cheap.
- Gyroscope – analyze your metrics and get insights into mindset and behavior change
- Ha'You Fit – this is where Qi Gong, fitness and breath work meet. Gentle exercise that is fantastic with HIT.
- Hartig & Helling – an "extremely low-radiation baby monitor" that works through a very low analogue radio signal. Again, this is important regarding EMFs – see the section on EMFs for more.
- Histamine Intolerance Cookbook my cookbook – low-histamine and mostly low-carb recipes. Woohoo.
- Holden Qi Gong – Jump-Start Your Qi Gong Practice with Easy Online Classes. Qi Gong is one of the best ways to activate your parasympathetic nervous system.
- HRV4Training – this app tracks your HRV daily and follows your parasympathetic nervous system activity over time, providing some great stats. My HRV levels and stress/histamine levels seem to be linked.
- Instant Heart Rate – this app claims to be the "most accurate mobile heart rate monitor". It showed me how certain foods would spike my heart rate super high – for instance, prawns. I don't (thankfully) need this app much anymore as it's been a long time since I've eaten prawns. Not every high-histamine food pushes my heart rate up, but it might be helpful for you to look at.

- Instant Pot – this is helpful for anyone with histamine intolerance, as previously discussed. It is a healthy, quick pressure cooker that allows you to cook low-histamine dishes. It cooks, steams, sautés, makes (histamine-intolerance-friendly) yogurts, and much more besides.
- James Nestor breath resources – an excellent collection of breathwork videos in one place.
- Joovv – an infrared light company. They are so serious about what they do, they've teamed up with the athletes of the San Francisco 49ers to help their recovery regime. I love this. Many of my followers on The Histamine Intolerance Site have had great success with red light therapy.
- Magnesium Breakthrough – for better sleep and looser joints. As mentioned above, I find it is good for my histamine intolerance.
- Night Shift mode – on the iPhone (Android and Kindle have similar options), which makes the phone a warmer hue in the evening. If you haven't enabled these on your devices, I recommend them for better sleep.
- Othership – a breathwork app that is good for de-stressing. I love this app – it's great for the rest-and-digest feeling we are aiming for in Chapter 5: *Low-Histamine Mindset.*
- Oura Ring – this tracks sleep quality, heart rate, heart rate variability, body temperature, respiratory rate, exercise, and lots more. This is useful from a histamine perspective as well as overall health.
- Readwise – is my book one of many books you've read on histamine intolerance? Perhaps you need to keep all your precious notes in one place. This syncs up with your Kindle highlights and sends you a daily

email. You choose how many quotes you get a day. I find it helpful to get daily reminders on my favorite books long after the original reading.

- SafeSleeve – this provides protection on your phone while you're holding it to your ear.
- Sam Harris's Waking Up app – for daily 10 or 20-minute meditations.
- Seeking Health Vitamin D – for immunity and health, especially in winter. This is another one of my regular supplements.
- SelfDecode – genetic testing and analysis, which is often useful with histamine intolerance. It also has some valuable articles on histamine intolerance.
- Sensate meditation pebble – this is potentially helpful for histamine intolerance sufferers who want to reduce their stress.
- Sleep Cycle – a free sleep app. Give yourself enough time to heal at night. This is an addictive geek out on sleep stats.
- Soleil Toujours – a non-toxic mineral sunscreen that doesn't make you look like a clown.
- Strategene – this strategic genetic testing option also analyzes DNA and gene results. There are specific histamine intolerance results on this site, which I recommend along with a good practitioner to help you interpret them.
- The Complete Guide To Fasting – I find intermittent fasting helps with histamine intolerance, but that's just me. Ask your practitioner.
- The Histamine Intolerance Masterclass – you may already have visited my site. Now go deep and take my Masterclass, complete with in-depth video lessons hosted by me.

- The Wand – described as "A Wine Filter That Removes Histamines & Sulfite Preservatives". It didn't work for me, but thousands say it does. If you still want to drink wine, then you could try this.
- Theragun – this is an incredible percussive massage tool, that is extraordinarily effective in easing away aches. Beware of cheap imitations; as I can tell you from experience – they don't work.
- Think Dirty – this app helps us discover potential toxins in household, personal care and beauty products. Use Think Dirty, EWG's Skin Deep or similar (like Yuka) to check cosmetic products for ingredients in a simple, non-confusing way.
- Ullo – this is another product that claims to remove sulfites from wine. It helps alleviate your sore head the next day. Again, you can try this if you want to drink wine while histamine intolerant, but ideally you would pause your alcohol intake to see how your symptoms improve.
- Una Mattress – certified organic materials from the groves of Hevea trees, with no smelly petrochemicals, and no fire-retardant chemicals. VOCs are an important consideration with histamine and mold issues.
- Veristable – monitor your glucose levels, rediscover nutrition, and determine what works for you. It's a great product, but not cheap.

11. 30-Day Histamine Intolerance Symptom Tracker

Use this tracker to monitor your symptoms, potential triggers, and progress. It's a valuable tool that can help you better understand your body's responses, and (most importantly) this could be an excellent way to share accurate information with your healthcare practitioner.

Categories

- Food/Drink Intake: remember to include everything you've eaten and drunk. Note any new foods, drinks or supplements here too.
- Symptoms: list all symptoms you've experienced.
- Symptom score: give your overall symptoms a score – 1 for worst, and 10 for best.
- Stress score: did you spend 13 hours in front of your laptop, or did you spend the day off relaxing with your family in the sunshine?
- Self-care: what did you do to look after yourself today? Jot it down – this is valuable information.
- Notes and thoughts: possibly the most important section. When you come back to analyze your metrics in the future (perhaps years in the future), what might be helpful to know about what you are experiencing or changing right now?

Bear in mind that everyone's experience with histamine intolerance is unique. What triggers a reaction in one person may not affect another person in the same way. This tracker is a tool designed to help you better understand your own body and needs. It's always important to consult with a healthcare professional regarding your symptoms and treatment options; this is designed to help you do that.

Day	Food / Drink	Symptoms	Symptom score (1 worst, 10 best)	Stress score (1 worst, 10 best)	Self care (eg exercise/ medita-tion)	Notes and thoughts
1						
2						
3						
4						
5						
6						
7						
8						
9						
10						
11						
12						
13						
14						
15						
16						
17						
18						
19						
20						
21						
22						
23						
24						
25						
26						
27						

28						
29						
30						

DATE

OVERALL SYMPTOMS (1 worst, 10 best)
HEADACHE (1 worst, 10 best)
GUT (1 worst, 10 best)
INFLAMMATION (1 worst, 10 best)
ENERGY (1 worst, 10 best)
EXERCISE (yes/no)
10 MIN MEDITATION (yes/no)
SUSPECT FOODS EATEN (list)
NOTES

A word on cooking and recipes

If you'd like to get stuck into low histamine recipes for every occasion, then please do check out my cookbook. It's er, originally entitled, *Histamine Intolerance Cookbook*.

This title was originally published under my company name, Ketoko Guides, all the way back in 2019. This was a name we adopted for a specialized series of health books. The idea was to allow me to work with a small, extremely talented team and specifically address an audience interested in health and nutrition.

And the books worked. They were very popular. There was only one problem with Ketoko Guides. Everyone knew it was me behind the books. The histamine intolerance world is small, and after all I made no secret of the fact that I'd published it with my talented team. So who was I trying to kid?

So now The Histamine Intolerance Cookbook is proudly published in my name. You'll notice each ingredient in that book has a (L) or a (M) by it. This corresponds to whether it is listed as a low-histamine or a medium histamine food in my food list. Actually you won't find any (H) ingredients in the recipes themselves, but I note some high-histamine foods along the way. I hope you'll find how varied and enjoyable eating low-histamine can be.

Finally, remember to consult with a healthcare professional when making dietary changes. Individual histamine tolerances do vary. Honestly, I must sound like a broken record. I know I've said this a million times in this book, but with histamine intolerance, it's real, so please take note.)

PART 4:

THE ONGOING JOURNEY

12. So you've got to the end of this book? What now?

"So, has anyone ever managed to heal to the point where they can once more eat, say, a nice Italian dinner out with their friends? Or a fun al fresco lunch at a Mexican restaurant? Or are we really looking at the rest of our lives subbing pumpkin for tomato sauce, never having a nice glass of wine again, forget about guacamole or a margarita?"

Suzanne, by email

The good news? Absolutely – many, many people heal fully and go back to enjoying those nice Italian dinners and fun Mexican lunches. That's exactly our goal here. This 30-Day Program isn't just about small changes; it's about setting the stage for a full healing journey. The path to reintroduction is not only possible, it's what we anticipate with the right steps and guidance.

Long-term Healing Strategies

As I've emphasized throughout, the real game-changer is tackling the root cause of histamine issues. It's often not a quick fix – it's certainly been a journey for me – and you'll likely need a functional medicine specialist to navigate some tests. As I replied to the email, the goal is total healing and reintroduction. Though it might be more about savoring one margarita instead of ten, it all depends on you and your journey!

The occasional margarita is now very much on the menu for me, although I'm strangely less bothered about it than I used to be. It is true to say that, on this journey, I've been lucky enough to speak to authorities in the field like Dr. Janice Joneja and Beth O'Hara, who've emphasized that they follow some version of a low-histamine diet on a long-term basis. They've found what works for them with their unique physiology and started to truly heal. I hope you will, too.

Day-to-Day Management

I still use the diet list in this book almost daily, and I encourage you to dive into the Low-Histamine Survival Kit that follows. The main thing is to try not to obsess – difficult, I know, with endless lists of suspect foods.

As your healing progresses, the goal is to worry less about each specific ingredient. Honestly, life works better when we're not obsessing!

We do cook mostly low-histamine at home (my wife Faith is used to substituting various ingredients when it's her turn to cook). But honestly, I feel so much better now that I can tolerate some high-histamine ingredients. I have a sweet tooth and have discovered that one particular brand of chocolate (Ritter Sport) doesn't seem to spike my histamine levels at all. It's hard to resist after having gone without for several years. Although, yes, I still sub in pumpkin for tomatoes, and I sort of prefer it.

I wish you great success on your ongoing journey to overcoming histamine intolerance. And our journey doesn't end here. Come and say hello at www.histamineintolerance. net and sign up for my regular newsletter where I cover all the latest advancements in the field.

NEXT STEPS

Please come and say hello at The Histamine Intolerance Site (www.histamineintolerance.net) with what you like and what you'd change in this book. I'm going to keep updating it with any new information as it becomes available. I hope you feel healthy and happy going low-histamine, and I wish you the best on your healing journey.

For more content, check out my podcast Zestology, where I've interviewed lots of low-histamine experts like Beth O'Hara, Dr. Tina Peers, Dilly Kumar, and many more.

And why not come and take my signature health course combining my two specialist areas, histamine and mindset/NLP.

The Healthy AF Method (www.tonywrighton.com/healthy) teaches you to deeply relax and initiate healing by using extraordinary and powerful techniques to activate the parasympathetic nervous system. (Without this deep state of calm we can't properly heal - and that's a massive problem with histamine intolerance.)

On this program, I help people to immediately start to feel better and less anxious about their health. (I created it because I needed it!) Then in the 'Long-Term Transformation' section, engage in a profound shift encompassing environ-ment, behavior, capabilities, values, beliefs, and identity. Ensure lasting change through a complete lifestyle overhaul.

Finally, you'll find a supportive community and loads of hista-mine-based chat, as - surprise, surprise - a lot of people with histamine intolerance find stress is their number one trigger.

REFERENCES

Introduction

1 https://www.ncbi.nlm.nih.gov/pmc/articles/PMC7982139/

Part One

1 https://www.ncbi.nlm.nih.gov/pmc/articles/PMC7463562/

2 https://www.sciencedirect.com/science/article/pii/S00029165232280533

3 https://pubmed.ncbi.nlm.nih.gov/17490952/

4 https://ajcn.nutrition.org/article/S0002-9165(23)28053-3/fulltext#secsect0005

5 https://www.ncbi.nlm.nih.gov/pmc/articles/PMC6667364/

6 https://www.ncbi.nlm.nih.gov/pmc/articles/PMC6682924/?report=reader

7 https://www.healthgrades.com/right-care/allergies/histamine-intolerance

8 https://www.ncbi.nlm.nih.gov/pmc/articles/PMC8308327/

9 https://pubmed.ncbi.nlm.nih.gov/30836736/

10 https://www.ncbi.nlm.nih.gov/pmc/articles/PMC4711860/

11 https://link.springer.com/article/10.1007/BF03354071

12 https://pubmed.ncbi.nlm.nih.gov/30043558/

13 https://pubmed.ncbi.nlm.nih.gov/973560/

14 https://www.sciencedirect.com/science/article/abs/pii/
S00099120120005681

15 https://www.performanceinhealth.com.au/2021/05/25/
the-oestrogen-histamine-connection-is-histamine-affect-
ing-your-menstrual-health/

16 https://balance-menopause.com/uploads/2021/09/
Histamine-Intolerance-1.pdf

17 https://www.ncbi.nlm.nih.gov/pmc/articles/PMC8021898/

18 https://www.ijidonline.com/article/S1201-
9712(20)30732-3/fulltext

Part Two

1 https://www.ncbi.nlm.nih.gov/pmc/articles/PMC3389384/

2 https://www.ncbi.nlm.nih.gov/pmc/articles/PMC5417051/

3 https://www.jneurosci.org/content/41/30/6564

4 https://www.sciencedirect.com/science/article/abs/pii/
S0166432816304168

5 https://www.sciencedirect.com/science/article/abs/pii/
S0031938415301463
https://www.ncbi.nlm.nih.gov/books/NBK553141/

6 https://www.ncbi.nlm.nih.gov/books/NBK553141/

7 https://www.ukhypnosis.com/hypnosis-research-evidence/

8 https://www.sciencedaily.com/
releases/2014/06/140602101207.htm

9 https://www.sciencedirect.com/science/article/abs/pii/
S107839030300226X

10 https://journals.plos.org/plosone/article?id=10.1371/
journal.pone.0213995

11 https://www.ncbi.nlm.nih.gov/pmc/articles/PMC9638701/

12 https://wvutoday.wvu.edu/stories/2020/04/08/
wvu-rockefeller-neuroscience-institute-and-oura-health-
unveil-study-to-predict-the-outbreak-of-covid-19-in-
healthcare-professionals

13 https://www.who.int/news-room/fact-sheets/detail/
ambient-(outdoor)-air-quality-and-health

14 https://pubmed.ncbi.nlm.nih.gov/10226072/

15 https://www.elsevier.es/en-revista-allergologia-et-im-
munopathologia-105-articulo-the-allergy-tooth-
paste-case-report-S0301054608758713

16 https://pubmed.ncbi.nlm.nih.gov/17877753/

17 https://nutesla.com/wp-content/
uploads/2010/08/14987547-Disturbance-of-the-immune-
system-by-electromagnetic-fields.pdf

18 https://pubmed.ncbi.nlm.nih.gov/11737520/

19 https://pubmed.ncbi.nlm.nih.gov/10859662/

20 https://www.nature.com/articles/srep21774

21 https://www.e-cep.org/journal/view.php?doi=10.3345/
cep.2019.01494

22 https://www.chm.bris.ac.uk/motm/histamine/jm/history.
htm

23 https://www.hopkinsmedicine.org/news/articles/2019/02/
hopkins-history-moments-3

24 https://www.frontiersin.org/articles/10.3389/
fphar.2018.00913/full

25 http://www.chm.bris.ac.uk/motm/histamine/c/antihista-
mines.htm

26 https://medlineplus.gov/druginfo/meds/a697038.html

27 https://www.annualreviews.org/doi/full/10.1146/annurev-
pharmtox-051921-084047

28 https://www.ncbi.nlm.nih.gov/pmc/articles/PMC5884427

29 https://www.epa.gov/report-environment/drinking-water

30 https://www.sciencedirect.com/science/article/pii/
S0013935120302784

31 https://www.sciencedirect.com/science/article/abs/pii/
S0923181118304547

32 https://www.ncbi.nlm.nih.gov/pmc/articles/PMC5448264/

33 https://onlinelibrary.wiley.com/doi/10.1111/jdv.13200

34 https://pubmed.ncbi.nlm.nih.gov/1371041/

35 https://pubmed.ncbi.nlm.nih.gov/27741023/

35 https://www.ncbi.nlm.nih.gov/pmc/articles/
   PMC9370036/#:~:text=Specialized%20pro-re-
   solving%20mediators%20

Made in the USA
Monee, IL
30 April 2024

57776064R00094